Āyurvedic Inheritance

A Reader's Companion

M S Valiathan
ChM FRCS FRCS(C) FRCP DSc (hc)
National Research Professor
Manipal University, Manipal, India

Routledge
Taylor & Francis Group
LONDON AND NEW YORK

MANIPAL
UNIVERSAL PRESS

First published 2024
by Routledge
4 Park Square, Milton Park, Abingdon, Oxon OX14 4RN

and by Routledge
605 Third Avenue, New York, NY 10158

Routledge is an imprint of the Taylor & Francis Group, an informa business

ISBN13: 9781032546216 (hbk)
ISBN13: 9781032546223 (pbk)
ISBN13: 9781003425830 (ebk)

DOI: 10.4324/9781003425830

Typeset in Cambria
by Manipal Universal Press - 576104

MANIPAL
UNIVERSAL PRESS

To

Caraka, Suśruta and Vāgbhaṭa

Whose trail shines undimmed despite the lapse of centuries

Transliteration chart

अ a	आ (ा) ā	इ (ि) i	ई (ी) ī	उ (ु) u	ऊ (ू) ū
ऋ (ृ) ṛ	ॠ (ॄ) ṝ	ऌ (ॢ) ḷ	ॡ (ॣ) ḹ		
ऎ e*	ए (े) e/ē*	ऐ (ै) ai	ऒ o*	ओ (ो) o/ō*	औ (ौ) au
अं (ं) ṃ	अँ (ँ) m̐	अः (ः) ḥ	ஃ ḵ		
क् k क़ q	ख् kh ख़ qh	ग् g ग़ ġ	घ् gh	ङ् ṅ	
च् c	छ् ch	ज् j ज़/ஜ z	झ् jh	ञ् ñ	
ट् ṭ	ठ् ṭh	ड् ḍ ड़ ḏ	ढ् ḍh ढ़	ण् ṇ	
त् t	थ् th	द् d	ध् dh	न् n	ഩ ṉ
प् p	फ् ph फ़/ஃப f	ब् b	भ् bh	म् m	
य् y य़ ẏ	र् r ऱ/ற/ற் ṟ	ल् l	ळ् ḻ ऴ/ழ/ழ் ĺ	व् v	ऽ :’
श् ś	ष् ṣ	स् s	ह् h	क्ष kṣ	ज्ञ jñ

क् (k), क (ka), का (kā), कि (ki), की (kī), कु (ku), कू (kū), कृ (kṛ), कॄ (kṝ), कॢ (kḷ), कॣ (kḹ), के (ke/kē), कै (kai), को (ko/kō), कौ (kau), कं (kaṃ), कः (kaḥ)

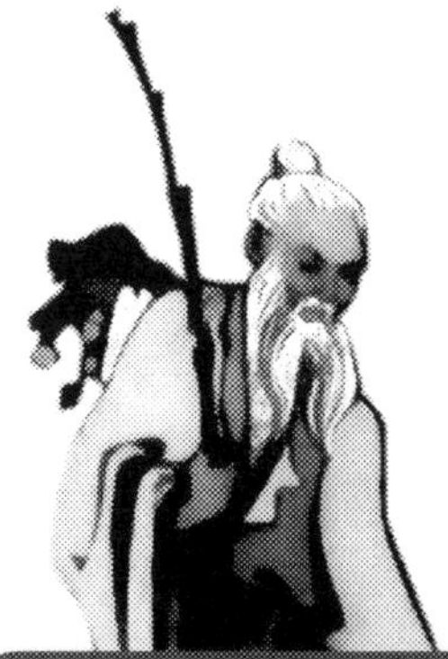

PREFACE

In 2015, I was privileged to record a course of video lectures on "India's Āyurvedic Inheritance" for the National Programme on Technology Enhanced Learning (NPTEL), which has achieved great success in providing over 800 high quality, open access video lecture courses for the students in our engineering colleges. This book is based on the general plan of my lectures but differs in contents and style. Its title harks back to the traditional Indian concept of four aspects of lifelong learning. These were instruction by the teacher, individual effort, learning from companions and lastly, wisdom gathered over a life time. The present book, it is hoped, may become a companion in Āyurvedic studies.

I am grateful to NPTEL authorities especially Professor Mangala Sunder Krishnan of the Indian Institute of Technology (IIT), Chennai for the support extended to me throughout my happy association with them and for endorsing the publication of this book. A word of thanks is due to Shri Madhu Reddy of Universities Press and Orient Blackswan Limited for permitting the use of many illustrations in this book from my three volumes on Caraka, Suśruta, and Vāgbhaṭa published by them in the last decade. I am greatly indebted to my wife, Ashima, for her support during the preparation and recording of the NPTEL lectures and the writing of this book.

It is a pleasure to thank Dr Ramdas M Pai, Chancellor of the Manipal University, who has encouraged me for the past many years in my literary endeavour in the congenial academic environment of the University. Manipal University Press (MUP) is one of the youngest and precocious institutions of the University, which has grown rapidly under the leadership of Dr Vinod Bhat, Vice Chancellor, Manipal University, Manipal and Dr Neeta Inamdar, Professor and Head, Department of European Studies (DES) and Chief Editor of MUP. I would extend my sincere appreciation to them for welcoming the publication of this book. Also, I would like to thank Professor Prabhakar Sastri for his masterly role in its critical editing. Ms Usha Kamath has not only typed the manuscript and its revisions with admirable skill and patience but also, made it ready for the publisher as she did for my four earlier books on Āyurveda. I am very thankful to her for her unfailing efficiency and devotion to work.

M S Valiathan

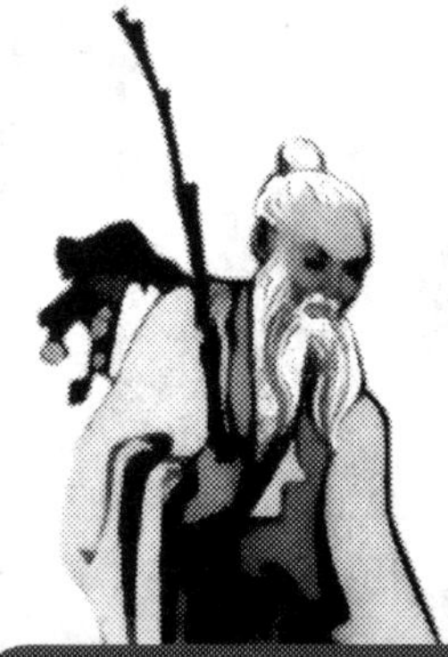

CONTENTS

1. Roots of Āyurveda 1
2. Traditional Medicine in Buddhist India 12
3. Evolution of Āyurveda from Caraka to Vāgbhaṭa 29
4. Philosophical Ideas in Āyurveda 38
5. Body in Health 50
6. Body in Disease 68
7. Food and Drinks 81
8. A Code For Living 100
9. Clinical Medicine 110
10. Medical Treatment of Diseases 120
11. Drugs (Dravyas) and Taste (Rasa) 131
12. Surgical Treatment of Diseases 141
13. Treatment of Fractures; Selected Surgical Procedures 161
14. Rejuvenation (Rasāyana) and Enhancement of Sexual Potency (Vājīkaraṇa) 175
15. Training of A Physician 183
16. A Science Initiative in Āyurveda (ASIIA) 195
17. Musings on Āyurveda 203
18. Quotations 217

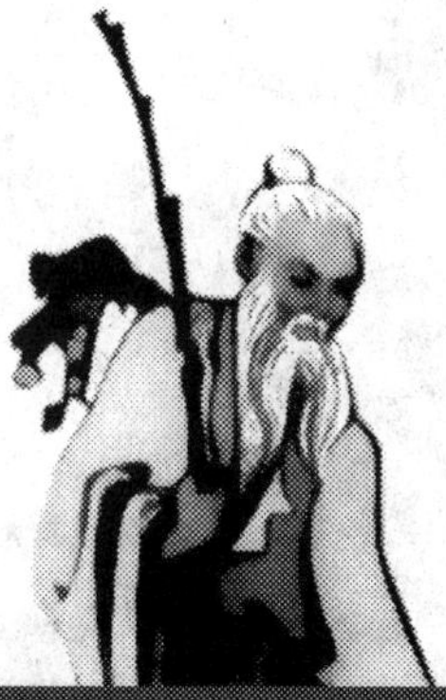

ACRONYMS

AH	Aṣṭāṅgahṛdaya
AN	Anguttara Nikāya
AS	Aṣṭāṅga Samgraha / Aṣṭāñga Saṅgraha
AV	Atharvaveda
BCE	Before Current Era
BG	Bhagavaḍ Gita
CE	Current Era
CS	Caraka Samhitā
DN	Digha Nikāya
DP	Dhammapada
J	Jātaka
MN	Majjhima Nikāya
MP	Milindapanho
SN	Samyutta Nikāya
SS	Suśruta Samhitā
VM	Viśuddhimagga of Buddhaghoṣa
VP	Vinayapiṭaka (especially Mahāvagga)

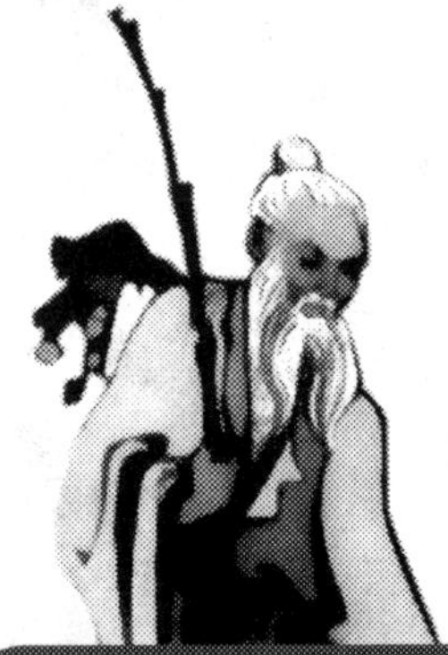

LIST OF FIGURES

Chapter 1: Roots of Āyurveda

Fig. 1: Mohenjo-Daro 3

Fig. 2: Treatment of Jaundice (Atharvaveda) 5

Fig. 3: Caraka 6

Chapter 2: Traditional Medicine in Buddhist India

Fig. 1: A deeply troubled Ajathaśathru taken to the Buddha by Jīvaka 15

Chapter 3: Evolution of Āyurveda from Caraka to Vāgbhaṭa

Fig. 1: References to infectious diseases and infected conditions 32

Fig. 2: References to non-infectious diseases 32

Chapter 4: Philosophical Ideas in Āyurveda

Fig. 1: Evolution (pariṇāma) according to Caraka 44

Chapter 5: Body in Health

Fig. 1: Course of Āhāra Rasa 61

Fig. 2: Origin of Tridoṣa 63

Chapter 6: Body in Disease

Fig. 1: Man in a pit 69

Chapter 8: A Code for Living

Fig. 1: Ādāna and Visarga (Dry and wet halves of the year) 105

Chapter 10: Medical Treatment of Diseases

Fig. 1: House for Treatment 122

Fig. 2: Jentaka (Chamber fomentation): Note the raised location on the bank of a lake and the central chimney; patient was placed in the circular space around the chimney. 122

Chapter 12: Surgical Treatment of Diseases

Fig. 1: Kāśirāja Divodāsa with seven disciples, Suśruta in the middle 141

Fig. 2: Basic Surgical Procedures: 145-146

i. Excision (chhedya)
ii. Incision (bhedya)
iii. Scraping (lekhya)
iv. Puncture (vedhya)
v. Probing (eṣya)
vi. Extraction (āhārya)
vii. Suturing (sīvya)

Fig. 3: Bandages: 147-148

i. Sheath bandage for amputated limb (kośa)
ii. Long roll for limbs (dāma)
iii. Cross like (svastika) for palm
iv. Four-tailed (khaṭvā) for head and neck
v. Circular (vibandha) for fracture ribs with moving chest
vi. Canopy like (vitāna) for protecting scalp wounds
vii. String (gosphaṇā) for nasal repair; often mentioned
viii. Five-tailed (pañcāṅgī); for nasal and facial injuries.

Fig. 4: Blunt Instruments: Forceps (Svastika): Examples (Named after animals) for removal of foreign bodies 151

i. Lion forceps (simhamukha)
ii. Tiger forceps (vyāghṛamukha)
iii. Wolf forceps (vṛkamukha)

Fig. 5: Forceps (Svastika): Examples (Named after birds) for removal of foreign bodies from depth 152

i. Crow forceps (kākamukha)
ii. Heron forceps (kankamukha)
iii. Osprey forceps (kurāramukha)

Fig. 6: Pincher forceps (Sandamśa) 153

i. With arms
ii. Without arms

Fig. 7: Spoon-shaped instrument (Tālayantra) 153

i. Single blade (ekatala)
ii. Double blade (dvitala)
Fig. 8: Tubular Instruments (Nādīyantra) 153
Examples:
i. Proctoscope (anal fistula)
ii. Rectal cannula for enema
Fig. 9: Rod like instruments (Śalāka) 153
i. Snake hood - like (sarpaphanamukha)
ii. Fish-hook like (badiśamukha)
Fig. 10: Sharp Instruments (śastr̥as) 154
i. Round tipped knife (maṇḍalāgra)
ii. Phlebotome (utpalapatra)
iii. Hand-held saw (karapatra)
iv. Straight tipped scalpel (vr̥ddhipatra)
v. Mouth like śarāri bird (śarārimukha)
vi. Sūci (Straight, Half and Full curved)
Fig. 11: Instruments for venesection 155
i. Horn (śr̥ṅga) for cupping
ii. Gourd (alābu)

Chapter 13: Treatment of Fractures; selected surgical procedures
Fig. 1 – 10: Fractures: 162-163
1. Karkaṭaka
2. Aśvakarṇa
3. Cūrṇita
4. Pichita
5. Asthichalita
6. Kāṇḍabhagna
7. Majjānugata
8. Atipātita
9. Vakra
10. Sphuṭita
Fig. 11: A bark splint (upayantr̥a) 164
Fig. 12: Fracture bed (kapāṭaśayana) 164
i. For leg bone
ii. For thigh bone
Fig. 13: Reconstruction of the nose 166
i. Nasal defect

ii. Flap from adjacent cheek turned to reconstruct the nose. Note the tubes inserted to keep nasal orifices open.

Fig. 14: Rectum; folds and chambers; arrows point to the folds and change in the direction of flow 169

Fig. 15: PC Ray 173

Chapter 15: Training of a Physician

Fig. 1: Vāgbhaṭa with disciples: Note that Vāgbhaṭa, a Buddhist, does not wear a holy thread 184

Fig. 2: Ācārya administering the oath on initiation, to a medical trainee before the sacrificial fire as witness and learned assembly 187

Fig. 3: One winged bird 190

Chapter 16: A Science Initiative in Āyurveda (ASIIA)

Fig. 1: Garcia da Orta 197

Fig. 2: Van Rheede 197

Fig. 3: Plants from Hortus Malabaricus 197

Fig. 4: Sir RN Chopra 197

Fig. 5: Towards Āyurvedic Biology 198

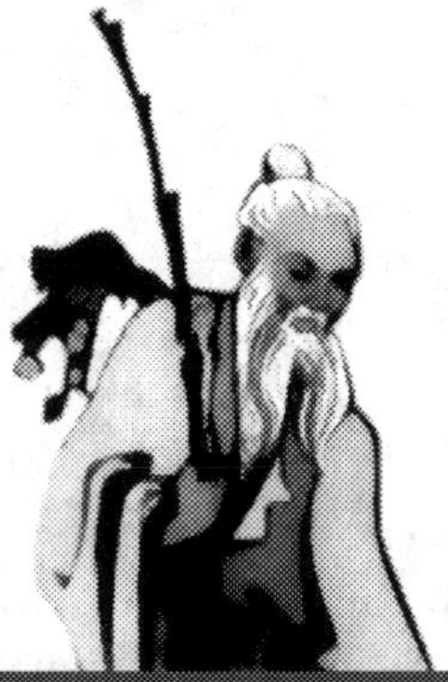

CHAPTER 1

Roots of Āyurveda

Folklore is a good place to begin the search for roots because it is a rich source of native wisdom and offers many clues to new discoveries. Known as "Lokavidyā" in India, it covers the entire gamut of human endeavour – agriculture, cottage industry, forestry, and of course, the practice of medicine. The extraction of precious discoveries from the vast quarries of folklore results from observations, which cast a spell on the mind of a genius. The observations may have been open to all, but few would have seen, let alone taken note of them. A classic example of the triumph of sourcing great discoveries from folklore is the story of vaccination in the 18th century. Edward Jenner qualified in medicine and set up practice in Gloucestershire in England where small pox epidemics were common and dreaded. He had an enquiring mind and used to be in regular touch with his mentor, John Hunter, in London who was a pioneer of scientific methods in surgery. Jenner found himself helpless in dealing with smallpox and was unimpressed by the spurious remedies being peddled by the physicians. However, he was surprised to hear from illiterate milkmaids that they were immune from small pox because they had suffered from "cowpox" earlier. This observation had been common knowledge for centuries but neither the public nor physicians had paid it the slightest attention. They dismissed the milkmaids' observation as unworthy of investigation. Jenner, on the other hand, was reminded of Hunter's admonition in a similar context "Why think? Why not experiment?" That inspired him to vaccinate subjects with cowpox material and make the epochal discovery of vaccination. Had he failed to pay attention like his contemporary physicians to traditional knowledge, which was freely available in the community, he too would have missed one of the most altruistic contributions to preventive medicine in history.

Āyurveda is the traditional medicine of India, which had been in vogue before the advent of the Buddha. A lot in Āyurveda has evolved from folk medicine in India as

Caraka – the highest authority in Āyurveda – recommends "shepherds and forest dwellers" among the teachers for students of medicine. This is not surprising because the urge to heal is as old as life. The broken chain of DNA tends to repair itself; wounds of the body tend to heal on their own; and animals, when sick, spot plants to chew and get well. This animal behaviour was noticed even in ancient times when a hymn in the Atharvaveda (AV) sought the protection of herbs as follows:

> I call upon those healing creepers known by pigs, mongoose, snakes, and Gandharvas to protect us. I call upon the healing herbs of the Aṅgirasas known by kites, divine herbs known by raghats (probably bees) and the plants known by swans to protect us.

This quote shows AV had recognized that animals and birds seek to heal themselves and know where to find help for self-medication. While the antiquity of Āyurveda is beyond doubt, we have intimations of public health even in the pre-history of India! Even before written texts appeared, unwritten traditions in public health existed in the Indian sub-continent. This is known from the spectacular examples of urban planning, dwelling units, drains, toilets, and baths in Mohenjo-Daro, Harappa, and many other sites spread across vast areas in Pakistan and India (Figure 1). This ancient civilization known after the Indus Valley – Sarasvatī is attributed to 3000-2500 BCE.[1] The tell-tale examples of public health engineering in the Indus Valley would suggest that the population had prior experience of epidemics and disease outbreaks because, preventive measures of public health follow long after a community experiences recurrent outbreaks of diseases, and discovers the clues for prevention in non-medical means such as sanitation, supply of clean drinking water, and proper housing. Unfortunately, we know too little about the pattern of diseases and medical traditions of the people of the Indus Valley – Sarasvatī civilization. We may know more when the Indus Valley script is finally deciphered.

Āyurveda; *its journey from Atharvaveda (AV):* According to Suśruta, Āyurveda is an "upāṅga" – of AV and originally had 100,000 verses composed by Brahma.[2] Upāṅga is a small part of an organ of the entire body of AV. It consists of six thousand verses and one thousand prose lines. Caraka characterised Āyurveda as a distinct Veda, which he ranked higher than the other Vedas because it safeguards life, without which no blessings would accrue in this life or the next. On the subject of medicine, which forms the core of Āyurveda, Caraka took the view that there was never a time when life did not exist or when thoughtful people did not exist; nor was there a time when medicines did not work on the body as indicated in Āyurveda. Āyurveda did not emerge at a specific moment out of nothing, but there was always a continuity in the science of life. When one talks of a beginning, it is merely a reference to the first systematized arrangement or text for instruction in Āyurveda.[3]

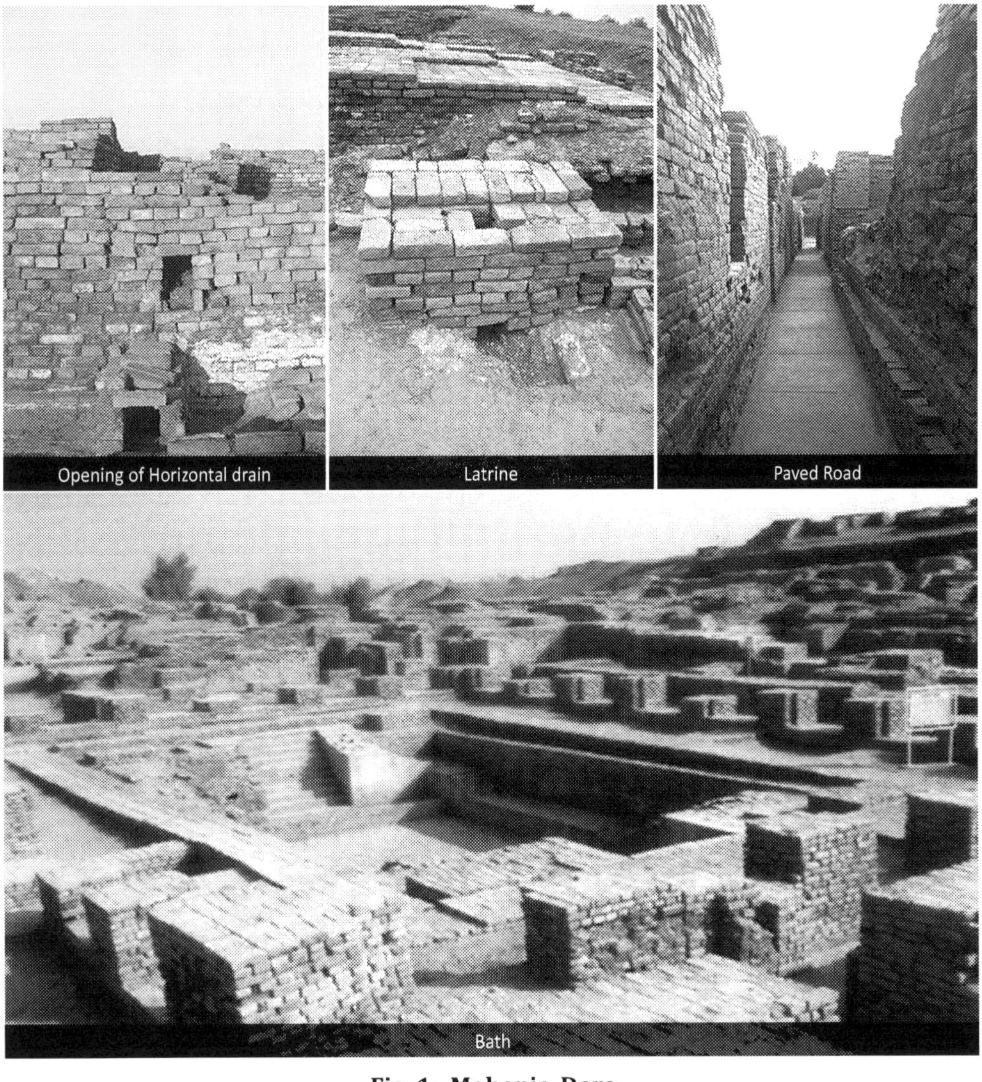

Fig. 1: Mohenjo-Daro

Vāgbhaṭa called Āyurveda an upaveda of the AV.[4] A commentator added that Āyurveda was one of the four upavedas of AV, the others being Dhanurveda, Gāndharvaveda, and Arthaśāstra. These references suggest that Āyurveda is probably as ancient as Vedas and had a special linkage with AV because they shared a profound concern for those suffering from diseases and the measures to alleviate the suffering. However, the term "Āyurveda" was never used in the Vedas or Upaniṣads and its earliest use is found in the Mahābhārata. Among the eight branches of Āyurveda, bhūtavidyā finds mention in the Chāndogya upaniṣad.[5] AV refers to hundreds of physicians and thousands of herbal medications,[6] which clearly suggests that the practice of medicine was then widespread. The absence of the term Āyurveda in the Vedas or Buddhist literature does not therefore imply that the concepts and practices of Āyurveda or their forerunners did not exist in the Vedic or Buddhist period.

Caraka urged the students of Āyurveda to revere AV because it attached great importance to the treatment of diseases (cikitsā) by propitiatory hymns, sacrificial offerings, auspicious rituals, penance, fasting, and incantations. AV has a large number of hymns addressed to Indra, Agni, and Varuṇa for protection and relief from various diseases. Indeed, the treatment of diseases in the AV was not complete in the absence of propitiatory hymns and rituals. While Caraka urged loyalty to AV in the study of Āyurveda, the medical therapeutics in CS differed significantly from the practice of medicine in the AV. In the period of AV, a patient with jaundice in a village settlement would be seen by a "bhiṣak" as AV mentions "hundreds of bhiṣaks" in the community. The bhiṣak's ritual would begin by tying an amulet around the patient's wrist to the accompaniment of invocations. Then a cow, reddish brown in colour, would be washed and a few drops of the wash water sipped by the patient. Following this, he would be made to sit on a piece of bull skin fixed with a peg after the skin had been dipped in milk and anointed with ghee (Figure 2). He would then be given a drink of porridge made of turmeric and milk. Next, the porridge would be used to daub the whole body of the patient from head to foot and washed off. He would then be given a fermented drink, made to sit on a cot and repeat the following hymn after the bhiṣak:[7]

> Up to the sun shall go thy heartache and thy jaundice;
> in the colour of the red bull do we envelop thee.
>
> We envelop thee in red tints, unto long life.
> May this person go unscathed, and free of yellow colour
>
> The cows whose divinity is Rohiṇī, and the cow is red, remember.
> They who more over are themselves red in their every form
> and every strength do we envelope thee.
>
> Into the parrots, these are the birds, into the ropanakas,
> (probably thrush) do we put thy jaundice, and furthermore,
> into the haridravas do we put thy jaundice.

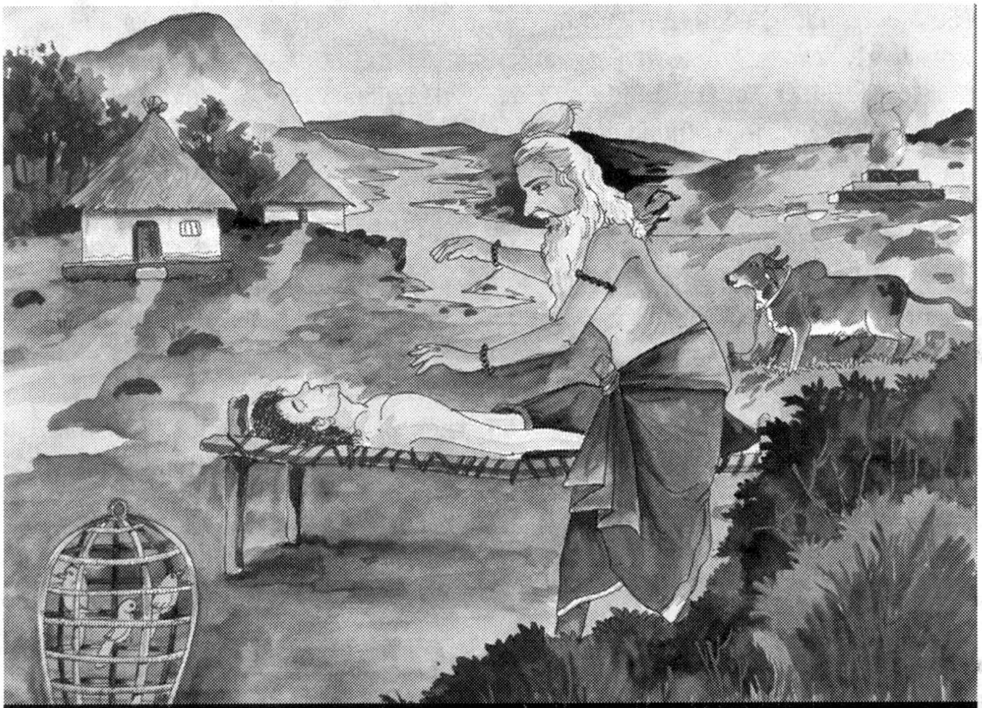

Patient on the cot; bhiṣak standing; yellow birds in a cage at the head and cow at the foot end of the cot

Fig. 2: Treatment of Jaundice (Atharvaveda)

The ritual was symbolic and the hymn held the key to unlocking the symbolism. The ritual implied the transfer of the patient's yellow colour to the yellow birds kept in a cage at the upper end of the cot as yellow was their natural colour; similarly, the cow's reddish brown colour would be transferred to the patient as natives of north-west India shared that colour. It was a widely-held belief in ancient India and other parts of the world that ailments of the body and mind could be transferred to other individuals or creatures by the use of charms and rituals. The porridge of turmeric consumed by the patient played no more than a small part of the ritual and its effect, it was believed, was brought about by supernatural forces and not pharmacologic action.

Fifteen or twenty centuries passed after AV when Caraka emerged, as he is acknowledged to have lived in the 1st century CE when Kaniṣka reigned over much of north India (Figure 3). Though reverential to AV, his approach to the treatment of jaundice was a study in contrast. Jaundice was well known to him and was called "Kāmala" in his famous Saṁhitā, which remains the foundational text of Āyurveda to this day. Kāmala was regarded as a manifestation of disturbed pitta in the gut and blood, and its evolution as a disease from premonitory to the terminal stage was clearly recognised. It was attributed mainly to the ingestion of inappropriate or incompatible food. The treatment consisted of dietary regimen, pañcakarma, and the intake of a variety of medicinal preparations, which were carefully selected by the physician. Gone were rituals and hymns, which was remarkable considering their central role in AV. This major break with Vedic tradition in the treatment of diseases was, in fact, not limited to jaundice. Caraka claimed explicitly that the practice of medicine had shifted from faith-based (daivavyapāśraya) of AV period to the reason-based (yuktivyapāśraya) mode in his time. While reason-based practice triumphed, it is a sobering thought that millions of people in India continue to demand and wear talisman and chant hymns to cope with life's many problems. This shows the hold of AV on the Indian mind! The powerful wind, which transformed the practice of medicine between AV and Caraka, was the reign of Buddhism, which will be discussed elsewhere.

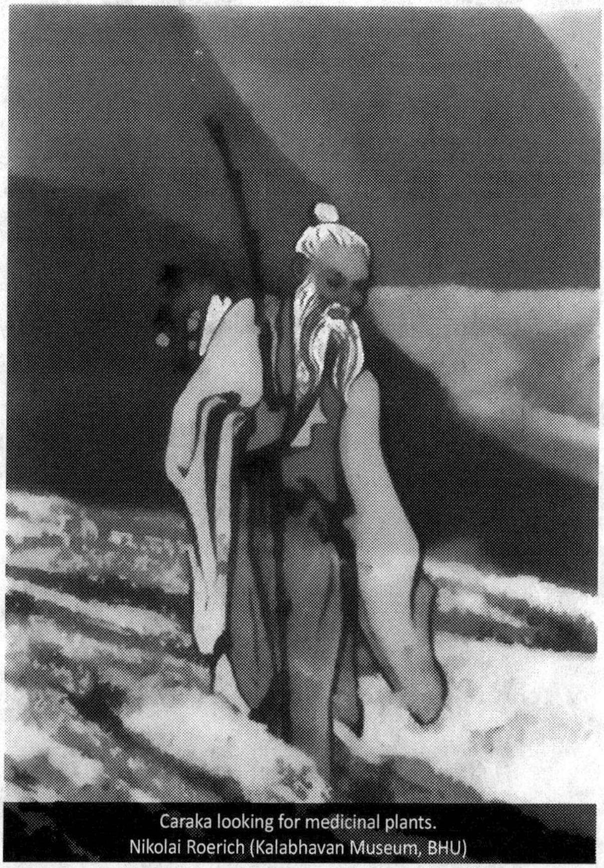

Caraka looking for medicinal plants.
Nikolai Roerich (Kalabhavan Museum, BHU)

Fig. 3: Caraka

The roots of current Āyurveda are traceable to elements of folk medicine, Atharvavedic tradition, and the traditional medicine practiced in Buddhist India.

Medicine in AV and Āyurveda: The transition from AV to Āyurveda in the practice of medicine took place over several centuries and was marked by change and continuity. Though a break in the practice of medical therapy is undeniable, a golden chain of many strands continued to link AV to Āyurveda despite the march of centuries. Consider the following links:

Organs and bones in the body: Table 1 lists a few parts and organs of the human body, from over 300 identified by Professor Filliozat in Vedic literature, especially the "Wonderful Structure of Man" of AV.

Table 1

Aṅga	Limb
Antapārśavya	Intercostal muscle
Antra	Entrails
Asṛj	Blood
Cakṣu	Eye
Dhamani	Vessel
Grīva	Neck
Guda	Rectum
Jaṭhara	Abdomen
Kanṭha	Throat
Lalāṭa	Forehead
Nāḍī	Canal, Vessel
Paṇi	Hand
Plīha	Spleen
Puritat	Pericardium
Snāvan	Tendon
Vasti	Urinary bladder
Vṛkka	Kidney
Hṛd	Heart

These terms were adopted by Caraka who also incorporated 360 bones, which had been totalled in AV. However, the meaning of some old terms had changed over the course of centuries such as "nāḍī" which was a conduit for air in AV became one for air and body fluids in Āyurveda.

Vital Functions: The chain of continuity does not consist of anatomy alone, but also involves motive functions of the body. In the Rig-Veda, wind in nature is regarded as the breath of gods; wind in the body - prāṇa – is looked upon as the motive power behind all movements in and of the body. According to this view, wind moves everything in nature; it is the life breath of gods and the humans. On death, human body would dissolve itself into nature and the wind - prāṇa – would be referred back to the wind in nature. This theme is echoed by Caraka and Suśruta when they speak of the "identification of the wind as the soul of the universe and the body." The Vedic idea of compartmentalising wind in the body into prāṇa, apāna, vyāna, samāna, and udāna is also found in Āyurveda. The attempt to identify the wind in nature with prāṇa in the body is of a piece with the Āyurvedic homology between the macrocosm and microcosm.

Medicinal Plants: The diverse strands of continuity are in display in the shared number of medicinal plants, which are mentioned in AV and Caraka Saṁhitā even though the mechanism of action of the plants was viewed very differently. While AV held that the action of medicinal plants in treating illness was brought about by supernatural forces, Āyurveda regarded the action in pharmacological terms.

Table 2: Examples of medicinal plants in Atharvaveda

Plant	Applications
Arkā	Enhances virility
Arjuna	For hereditary diseases
Añjana	For inflammations; heart disease
Apāmārga	Cleanses the body
Udumbara	Promotes strength; improves fertility
Māṣaparnī	Enhances virility
Kuṣṭha	Febrifuge
Bhṛngrāja	Improves complexion; promotes hair growth
Guggulu	Effective against vāta
Jīvantī	Promotes strength
Darbha	For snake bite
Daśamūla	Tonic following delivery
Pathyā	For treating injuries
Pippalī	Febrifuge; for vāta disorders
Pṛśniparṇī	For piles; female genital disorders
Vacā	Antidote to poison
Bilva	Antidote to snake poison
Priyaṅgu	Febrifuge
Śalaparṇī	For diseases of cattle
Soma	Effective against all diseases
Dāruharidrā	Effective against pallor; jaundice

Table 2 gives examples of medicinal plants mentioned in AV, which are currently used in Āyurveda. The hymns in AV were generally addressed to the plants to seek their protection from the wrath of gods or for their beneficence.

Attitude to Nature: The theme of continuity stands out again in the fundamental attitude of Atharvan hymns and Āyurvedic classics towards nature and human life. The Vedic attitude to earth, rivers, trees, birds, and natural phenomena such as dawn was always soaked in admiration and reverence. The grand hymn of AV – Bhūmisūkta – was an inspirational ode to earth, which intoned, "earth is my mother, I am her son". Here are other examples of Vedic hymns, which celebrate the splendour of nature:

> Within waters – I have heard from Soma – are all medicines that heal, and Agni, who blessed all.
> The waters contain all medicines.[8]

> Two bright winged Birds knit together; friends have found their home in the same tree.
> One of them eats the sweet pippala fruit; the other that does not eat, looks on.[9]

> At the entry and exit (from the house)
> Let the Dūrvā grow and flower
> Let a spring rise,
> and let a lake greet with lotuses in bloom.[10]

On a similar note, Ātreya's discussions with students, as reported by Caraka, were held in the Himalayan country of great natural beauty. His stipulations for building a house for patient's treatment included its location in a quiet and peaceful place, far from the madding crowd and vulgar displays, marked by shady trees in abundance, lakes with pellucid water, roaming cattle, and the space enlivened by bird song. There are many passages in the Great Three (Bṛhattrayī) of Āyurveda which brim with profound love of nature.

Attitude to Life: Above all, Vedic hymns and Āyurveda are united in their attitude toward life on earth, which is cheerful, lively, and joyful. Many a hymn in the Vedas sought life for a 100 years and a famous quote is the following:

> "Gods, may we, with our ears, listen to what is good,
> And, O Holy Ones! with our eyes see what is good;
> And may we, with firm limbs and bodies,
> offering hymns of praise to you,
> enjoy the divinely ordained term of life"[11]

Never was there any denigration of the body or disparagement of life, nor a whiff of world – renouncing asceticism in the Vedic panorama. Not only was the Āyurvedic attitude to life equally joyful and celebrant, two of the eight branches of Āyurveda were devoted to the promotion of healthy and pleasurable ageing (Rasāyana) and the enhancement of sexual potency and fecundity (vājīkaraṇa). Āyurveda acclaimed a full life enthusiastically while cautioning against the "non-use, overuse and misuse" of sense organs.

Āyurveda – a science of perennial healing: We began this chapter by noting that the urge to heal is as old as life itself. From an evolutionary point of view, life could not have survived, let alone evolved, in the absence of healing which was an evolutionary necessity. Practice of medicine, which emerged much later, could facilitate the healing process, which was innate and beginningless. Caraka claimed however, that Āyurveda is not only beginningless but is also endless because its province covers all that exists in nature, which are perennial. He noted that pleasure and pain, health and ill health, causes and symptoms of disease, and their interactions are never-ending. Secondly, therapeutic substances possessing properties such as heavy/light and cold/hot obey the law of increase and decrease by similarity and dissimilarity (śamānya and viśeṣa) without end. Thirdly, the properties associated with each of the five bhūtas, which constitute the universe including the human body, are bound to each other eternally.[12] Therefore, so long as life is inseparable from health and disease, happiness and misery and so long as their manifold relationships remain endless, Āyurveda will flow forever as a perennial stream of healing.

Āyurveda *Today:* Tracing its roots to the Vedic period, Āyurveda had a long and uninterrupted history of learning and practice. It was however a chequered history. A brilliant start from the AV, growth with stabilisation and spread in India and abroad during the Buddhist period and the golden age of systematisation of the Bṛhattrayī were followed by a 1000 years of stagnation and decline for reasons which are not entirely clear. The lowest point was perhaps the end of the 19th century when the government was indifferent, if not hostile, to the practice of Āyurveda, and its own traditional Gurukulas and institutions had collapsed. A precarious survival was made possible by its inherent vitality, the patronage of common people and a few visionary leaders of Āyurveda who shone as lighthouses here and there in India in the course of a long night. A resurgence came after independence and steady gain in momentum. Āyurveda remains highly popular and millions of Indians especially in rural areas seek medical help from Āyurvedic physicians. More than two hundred Āyurvedic colleges graduate over 20,000 physicians every year and three universities and Institutes provide postgraduate training and facilities for research. Research in Āyurvedic drugs are pursued in Central Universities, National Laboratories and Industry, which accounts for the annual production of Rs 6000 crores. Āyurveda has a separate Ministry in the Government of India and enjoys strong support in the states where most of the Āyurvedic colleges and hospitals are located. The Central Ministry of AYUSH has a large number of developmental programmes including educational institutions, promotion of research through CCRAS, the Traditional Knowledge Data Library (TKDL), publication of the Āyurvedic pharmacopeia, the promotion of Āyurvedic education and training abroad by the establishment of Chairs in foreign universities, and the exchange of students and faculty. Internationally Āyurveda is recognised as Complementary and Integrative Medicine and Āyurvedic scholars are often sought to teach courses abroad. Apart from traditional research in herbal drugs, the Department of Science and Technology, Government of India, has recently set up a Task Force in Āyurvedic Biology, which supports research in modern biology based on cues from Āyurveda. Āyurveda marches on.

References:

1. RC Majumdar. *History and Culture of Indian People*. Bharatiya Vidya Bhavan, Mumbai. Vol. 1 Page 105.
2. *SS* Sūtra 1: 1 -5
3. *CS* Sūtra 30: 24
4. Aṣṭaṅga Saṅgraha Sūtra 1: 42
5. Ch. Upaniṣad VII. 1.2
6. *AV* 11: 9.3
7. Atharvaveda Tr. W. D. Whitney MLB Delhi 1996. Vol. 1: 1: 22 Page 821.
8. *AV* 1: 6.2
9. *AV* 1: 1.20
10. *AV* 6: 106.1
11. Ṛigveda 1: 89 - 8
12. *CS* Sūtra 30: 26 – 29

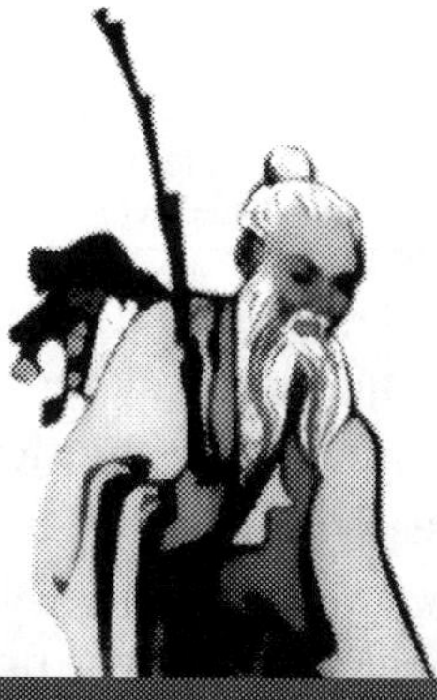

CHAPTER 2

Traditional Medicine in Buddhist India

Buddhist India: Buddha was born in or about 560 BCE in the ancient town of Kapilavastu in Nepal. At the age of 29, he made his "Great Renunciation" and after six years of struggle and severe austerities he attained supreme enlightenment. Thereafter, he spent over 40 years as an itinerant preaching a doctrine which drew millions to him. The influence of Buddha's teaching on the Indian mind and every aspect of life in India in succeeding centuries was stupendous and to quote Professor Dasgupta, "It is impossible to overestimate the debt that the philosophy, culture, and civilisation of India owe to it in all her developments for many succeeding centuries."[1] Buddha's compassion for the ill was so legendary and his insistence on maintaining good health was so strong that he was revered as a luminous sage who could sweep away illness from the body and mind. Vāgbhaṭa saluted him as the "un-preceded physician" (apūrvavaidya) in the invocatory verse of Aṣṭāṅgahṛdaya.

According to Rhys Davids, the earliest Buddhist records reveal that north India in the sixth and seventh centuries BCE consisted of a few powerful kingdoms and, side by side, a few republics which were independent in different degrees.[2] The kingdoms were Magadha with capital at Rajagaha, which figures prominently in Buddha's life, Kosala with capital at Savatthi, Vamsas with capital at Kosambi, and Avanti with capital at Ujjain. But political divisions, which were based on the names of people or tribes, blurred geographical divisions. At or shortly before the advent of Buddhism, 16 such political divisions had emerged such as Aṅga, Magadha, Kāśī, Malla, Kuru, Pañcāla, Gandhāra, etc. Gandhāra is of special interest because, it included the eastern districts of modern Afghanistan and north-west Punjab. Its capital was Takṣaśilā, which was the seat of a great university especially noted for medical studies. There are several stories of the medical training of Buddha's famous physician – Jīvaka – in Takṣaśilā. Other famous alumni attributed to Takṣaśilā include Pāṇini – the grammarian and Caraka.

Against the political and social background in India before the Buddha, it is necessary to understand the intellectual climate in that period of Indian history in view of its bearing on a physician's training and practice of medicine. According to Professor Dasgupta, three lines of thought dominated the philosophical climate: in the first place, Vedic sacrifices including the rituals of Atharvaveda (AV) could secure the desired results for an individual; secondly, the Upanishadic doctrine held that Brahman and self are identical and constitute the sole reality – everything else is unreal; and thirdly, a materialistic view (Lokāyata) that there is no abiding reality and everything results from a chance association of circumstances. Outside these three schools, yoga practices were prevalent but they had not graduated into a philosophical system. This was the intellectual climate where Buddhism broke in like a whirlwind upsetting many things. It questioned Vedic authority, overturned ancient beliefs, and wrecked the performance of sacrificial rituals including those for the practice of medicine. Over the centuries when Buddhism became the dominant faith in India, Āyurveda was championed by Buddhist physicians who fully shared the concern for suffering and the mission to provide relief, which characterised Āyurveda later.

Access to the medical tradition in Buddhist India: In attempting to study the practice of medicine between the Atharvaveda and Caraka, a serious difficulty is the non-availability, if not non-existence, of texts and documents, which directly deal with the subject. Carakasaṃhitā of the first century CE states that it was redacted from Agniveśatantra, which had been written by Agniveśa and had been a standard text for centuries earlier. Apparently Agniveśa was a disciple of Acharya Ātreya who asked his handful of disciples at the conclusion of their training to compose a medical text based on what they had learnt. All disciples complied and their texts were presented before an assembly chaired by Ātreya. Agniveśa's text was acclaimed as the best and it went on to claim authority until Caraka came to redact it after five or six centuries when Buddhism had established its intellectual and religious reign in India. The texts composed by some of the fellow disciples of Agniveśa – Hārīta and Bhela are available in part or full but their authenticity remains controversial. It is certain that Agniveśatantra existed because, apart from Caraka's acknowledgement, Cakrapānidatta of the 10th century CE who wrote the commentary Āyurveda Dīpika on Carakasaṃhitā quotes directly from Agniveśatantra. We are therefore obliged to depend on canonical Buddhist texts to learn medical history though they are primarily religious literature addressed to spiritual seekers. Many medical texts in Pāli language may have been written and studied between the rise of Buddhism in the fifth century BCE and the composition of Carakasaṃhitā in the first century CE, but they were lost or ignored because Pāli scholars became fewer and the Brahmin scholars may have been averse to study the books written by those who repudiated Vedic authority.

Professor Jyotir Mitra of Banaras Hindu University did a great service by writing his important book on Āyurvedic material in Buddhist literature based on a 10 year study of Āyurvedic texts of Caraka, Suśruta, Bhela, Kaśyapa, and Vāgbhaṭa and the Tripiṭaka literature of Buddhism. "Tripiṭaka" are Buddhist scriptures in Pāli consisting of Sutta (relating to doctrines), "Vinaya" (relating to the rules for the monks) and "Abhidhamma" (relating to the same subject as Sutta but treating them in scholastic and technical terms). "Tripiṭaka" are believed to consist of the original teachings of the Buddha. Another source of great value is Viśuddhimagga of Buddhaghosha (380–400 CE), which contains more accurate information on human anatomy than in Āyurveda. The other sources of Āyurvedic material in Buddhist literature are Milindapanho of considerable authority and philosophical value and Jātaka tales, which give a wealth of information on the social and economic conditions in ancient India, training of physicians in Takṣaśila, and the life and work of Buddha's physician, Jīvaka.

Buddha and Jīvaka: It is impossible to consider the practice of traditional medicine in Buddhist India without understanding the inspirational role of the Buddha who transformed the lives of millions of his contemporaries and successors. Jīvaka, on the other hand, was a gifted surgeon who was Buddha's physician, an ardent disciple, and benefactor of the Sangha.

Buddha's compassion knew no bounds and his concern for the ill and their recovery was so profound that he was revered as a "physician and surgeon (bhisako, sallakato)" by the common people. He worked no miracles – indeed he abhorred them - but the ill and suffering were comforted by his mere presence. In the Teviggasutta – among his earliest sayings – Buddha condemned a number of popular practices in healing as "low arts and lying practices." These included teaching spells to cure snake bites, to impart sexual potency or impotence, to relieve headache by applying ear drops, using collyrium, and so on. But when he found that some popular practices brought relief to patient's suffering, compassion softened his views on medical procedures. For example, he approved the use of animal fats (fish and swine) in preparing food, of chunnam for boils and scabies, of nasal speculum for inducing nasal purging, of bloodletting for intermittent fever, of salves, astringent decoctions, fumigation, and even excision of proud flesh in chronic ulcer, of purgatives for eliminating perturbed doṣas, of administering a decoction of cow dung as an emetic following the ingestion of poison, and several more. He permitted Jīvaka, his physician, to treat him without placing restrictions. He did forbid Bhikkus from undergoing surgery when the operation for anal fistula went terribly wrong in a Bhikku who suffered piteously. There is however no evidence that he forbade surgical procedures on the laity as Jīvaka continued to do surgery on kings including Bimbisara and commoners.

Jīvaka, Buddha's physician, was an extraordinary figure. An infant orphan found abandoned on the steps of King Bimbisara's palace in Pataliputra, he was brought up as a prince by Prince Abhaya who named him Jīvaka. As a teenager, he discovered that he was not a prince but had been an orphan. This steeled his resolve to scale professional heights and made him travel all the way to Takṣaśila for training as a physician. He was accepted as a student by Atreya on the basis of his brilliant performance at an interview. As he had gone on his own and not as a prince, he was too poor to pay his fees and worked part time by providing domestic service. He excelled in his studies and outperformed his classmates every time. The Jātaka tales have many interesting stories about Jīvaka's student days and class tests. He passed out triumphantly and earned a fortune by successfully treating a rich merchant's wife for her "incurable headache" by a nasya procedure on his way back home. Back in Pataliputra, his brilliance won royal attention and he became the physician to King Bimbisara. He was moved by Buddha's teaching and became his devoted disciple and physician. It is recorded that he carried out a trephining of the skull and removed two worms successfully from a gravely ill merchant who loaded him with gifts. It was typical of Jīvaka to receive large fees and gifts from his rich patients and donate them to the Sangha.

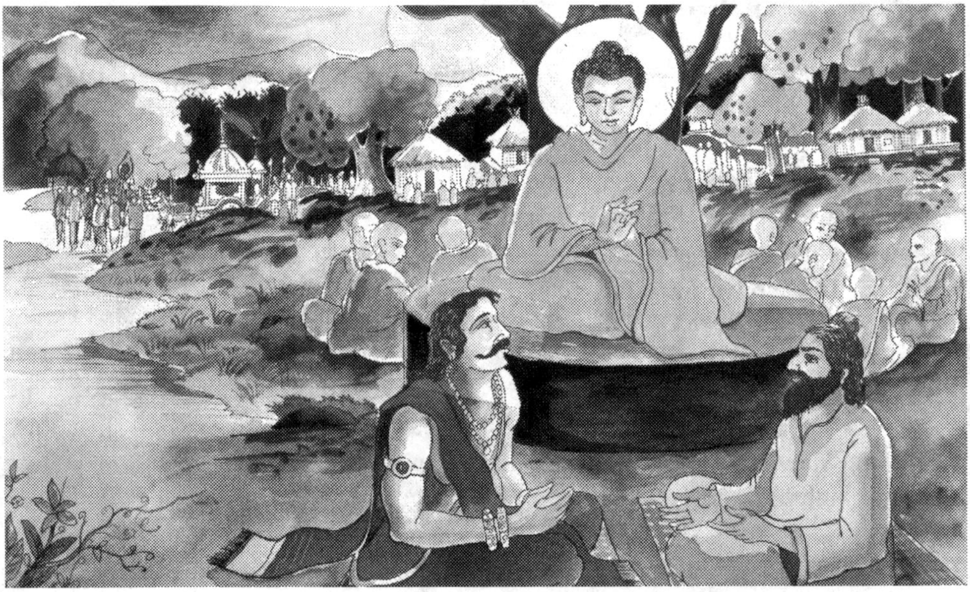

Fig. 1: A deeply troubled Ajathaśathru taken to the Buddha by Jīvaka

It is important to note that Suśrutasaṃhitā does not mention trephining of the skull even though many other surgical procedures are mentioned and described. This could be an indication that Suśruta lived before the time of Buddha and Jīvaka.

Traditional Medicine in Buddhist India; the forerunner of Āyurveda: It is a fact that none of the Buddhist texts use the term "Āyurveda." Whenever they refer to the practice of medicine, the term employed is "tikiccha." But there is enough evidence, as will be discussed below, that the basic concepts, ideas, medical procedures, and principles of practicing medicine in Āyurveda were anticipated, if not known and promoted, by the physicians and scholars of Buddhist India. These constituted the forerunner of Āyurveda, which expressed itself in the Carakasaṃhitā. Examples of medical knowledge and practices, which existed in Buddhist India and reflected in ancient Buddhist literature, are outlined below:

Basic concepts

The basic concepts are: Aṣṭāṅga, Pañcabhūta, and Tridoṣa.

Aṣṭāṅga: The Dīghanikāya[3] of sutta-piṭaka mentions five branches of medicine as follows:

- Vasakamma (Enhancement of sexual potency)
- Śālākya (Head and neck diseases)
- Sallakatiya (Surgery)
- Dāraka-tikiccha (Paediatrics)
- Mūlabhesajjānam (General Medicine)

There are ample references to bhūtavidyā (mental illness) and viṣavijja (poisoning) although they are not formally listed. Rasāyana is left out as living long with good health and vigour did not interest Buddhist sages who prized nirvāṇa. The eight divisions – kāyacikitsā (general medicine), śālākya (head and neck diseases), śalya (surgery), agada (poisoning), bhūtavidyā (mental illness, diseases caused by spirits), kaumārabhṛtya (paediatrics), rasāyana (rejuvenative medicine), and vājīkaraṇa (therapy by aphrodisiacs) of medicine are fundamental in Āyurveda.[4]

Pañcabhūta: The terms bhūta and dhātu appear in Buddhist literature and Āyurveda. Bhūta signifies ākāśa, vāyu (air), tejas (fire), ap (water), and pṛthvī (earth) and dhātu includes seven tissues of the body: rasa (chyle), rakta (blood), māṃsa (flesh), medhas (adipose tissue), asthi (bone), majja (marrow), and śukra (semen). There are subtle differences in the views of Buddhaghosha in VM and Caraka in the characteristics of bhūtas, mahabhūtas, and dhātus and their interpretation, but they remain readily identifiable. In the enumeration of bhūtas, VM stipulates four i.e., pṛthvī, ap, tejas, vāyu[5] whereas Majjahima Nikaya added ākāśa later and made the total of five bhutas.[6] In Āyurveda, bhūtas are fixed at five. There is much in common in the description of the characteristics of the five bhūtas in VM on the one hand and CS, and SS on the other.

Tridoṣa: The three doṣas – vāta, pitta, and kapha are mentioned frequently in Buddhist literature including the dialogues of the Buddha, VM, and MP. The properties of each doṣa are not discussed, but their derangement as a cause of disease and death is mentioned. According to the Buddha, the imbalance and balance of doṣas (sannipātikāni) are responsible for suffering and happiness in illness and health.[7] The causes which derange the three doṣas are listed in MP.[8]

In Āyurveda, tridoṣa became a central doctrine. Their balance or equilibrium (doṣasāmya) and imbalance or disequilibrium (doṣavaisāmya) are equivalent to health and ill health. Caraka and Suśruta who described the stages of illness differently as three and six tracked the stages from premonitory to the fully manifest stage.

Medical sciences

Anatomy: VM is a post-canonical work, which was written by a matchless scholar - Buddhaghoṣa. It is a repository of canonical teachings but also has the distinction of providing valuable descriptions of anatomy. The following are some of the highlights from VM and some other texts.

- The Anguttara Nikaya[9] quotes the Buddha's exhortation to the Bhikkus on the anatomical study of a leg in a cadaver. The technique described employed a rope of horse hair which was wound around the leg and tightened gradually until it cut through outer and inner skin, muscle, sinews, bones and bone marrow serially. This is obviously superior to agreeing with "warrior nobles, great Brāhmaṇas and great house holders."
- Body is a composed of four primary elements. It is full of filth of many kinds and a home of many diseases. It is shared by 80 families of worms colonizing on the outer and inner layers of the body. The worms take birth, grow old and die, evacuate, and make water, and use the body as a urinal, privy, maternity home, hospital, and charnel ground. Several hundred diseases find their home in it.[10]
- Body contains over 300 bones, 180 joints, and 900 ligaments; these are enveloped in 900 sheets of muscle and covered over with inner and outer skin with orifices at appropriate locations. The oozing from the orifices and the entire description is designed to create certain disgust towards the body.
- Corpses were classified into 10 types. Preservation of the body in oil was known.[11]

- Corpses were used as subjects for meditation.
- Buddhaghosha urged mindfulness in introspecting on the "32 aspects" of the body. These are various parts, organs, tissues, and fluids of the body from head to foot,[12] that are listed in great detail. Buddhaghoṣa's total of 300 bones agrees with Suśruta's and differs from Caraka's.

The anatomical descriptions have similarities with those in Suśruta but, like Āyurvedic classics of Suśruta and Caraka, they show no awareness of the function of the brain, lung, or kidney.

Physiology: The descriptions in physiology in VM are meagre and reveal a much earlier stage of understanding from that in the Carakasaṃhitā. For example, in discussing digestion, food and drinks are said to fall into the gut (mahāsrota) and get divided into five parts. The worms eat one part, fire in the stomach burns the second part, third becomes urine, fourth becomes faeces, and fifth part becomes nourishment for the body. Caraka's account of digestion shows a more advanced level of understanding including the role of stomach, duodenum, bile, intestine, and the transport of nutrient substances to the tissues.

Hygiene: Health was highly prized in Buddhist literature. The Dhammapada declared health as the highest gain.[13] Buddhism enjoined strict adherence to the principles of public health in the lives of Bhikkus and laity and gave instructions in great detail, which have no parallel in Āyurveda. Take, for example, the minute details in the construction, maintenance, and personal use of latrines.[14] The greatest attention was paid to personal hygiene of the users of latrines, who had to make sure it was left clean for the next user. Latrines were sheltered from cold and rain and had doors to ensure privacy. Special provision of chairs was made for the frail and elderly who sought to use the latrine. In comparison with such elaborate attention to latrine in Buddhist texts, Āyurveda is silent on this important topic. Vāgbhaṭa does refer to evacuation but his instructions were of a different kind altogether. For example, one should not defecate in public places such as cemetery, parks, beneath a tree, and on playgrounds, one should not face the sun and moon while relieving oneself, mind should be focused on defecation, etc. There was no mention of a latrine. The Buddha forbade open defecation.

Dental hygiene: Dentapoṇa was the name for a dental cleaner in Buddhist literature; but its source was not indicated.[15] Carakasaṃhitā, on the other hand, describes disposable dental cleaners made from the twigs of plants such as Karañja and Arjuna.

Regular brushing of the teeth was recommended and the advantages and disadvantages of not brushing were carefully listed in Vinayapiṭaka.[16] Caraka advised brushing twice a day and indicated its merits including removal of fetor and improvement of appetite.

Mosquito net: When mosquitoes harassed the monks, Buddha permitted them to use mosquito net. Mosquito nets are not mentioned in Āyurveda.

Purification of water: Water purification was known and recommended by the use of a gem (maṇi), which clears turbid and foul water on immersion.[17] Another method was the use of a strainer (parisāvana), which the Bhikkus in fact carried with their water pot. The strainer was apparently used to save the living things which water might have contained and not to protect the individual drinking the water.[18] To pollute water was a punishable crime and no one was permitted to ease in water.[19]

Personal conduct

Personal care: Detailed instructions were given in Buddhist literature as well as the texts of Caraka and Suśruta on regular hair-cut, special haircut, prohibition of hair dressing for monks, and on paring of nails.

Anointment: It is interesting that Buddhaghosha[20] found no merit in body anointment which is extolled in Āyurveda for a variety of benefits for the skin, complexion, and strength of tissues.[21] Surprisingly, he gives instructions on oiling the body perhaps as a concession to the demand of consumers!

Bath: Buddhist literature laid great stress on the guidelines for the construction of bathrooms as cleansing the body was regarded as supremely important. It would appear that bathrooms could either be regular bathrooms for cleaning the body with water, or could also be rooms for steam bath. There is evidence that steam baths were commonly used. The construction, maintenance and use of the bathrooms were described in exquisite detail. In the use of bathrooms, elders were always given preference. Nuns had separate bathrooms and they were forbidden from using the bathrooms for men or bathing against the current in a stream. Pools were also used for recreational bath, which were sometimes gifted to the Saṃgha by rich devotees. Special civil engineering techniques were used to provide the proper flooring and sides for the pool and pipes for drainage of stagnant water.[22]

Āyurvedic texts do commend the merits of bath but they do not go into the materials and methods for the construction, maintenance, and use of bathrooms.[23]

A survey of the practice of public health described in the Buddhist texts shows that the standards prescribed not only equalled those prescribed in Āyurveda but were also superior in some respects.

Food and drinks

In Buddhist literature, food is classified into four categories: soft (bhojanīya), hard (khādanīya), lickable (lehya), and beverages (peya).[24]

A few examples are given below:

Soft food: Five kinds; Boiled rice, boiled mixture of barley and beans, food made with flour, fish, and meat

Hard food: Five kinds; Roots, stalks, leaves, flowers, and fruits

Lickables (Lehya): Sādava, Pāyasa

Beverages (Peya): Fruit juice, wine

Food articles were categorised into:

i. Cereals and pulses;
ii. Dairy products; and
iii. Non-vegetarian food.

Cereals and pulses: Seven kinds of grains and seven kinds of pulses were the main items of staple food. Rice preparations were popular and their 10 merits were commended.[25] The pulses commonly used included mudga, māṣa, masūra, and kalāya.

Dairy products: Milk, curd, buttermilk, and ghee were used by monks and laity.

Non-vegetarian foods: People ate the meat of cow,[26] fowl, fish, lizard, crow, and bull. There was no prohibition of cow's meat. Buddha condemned animal sacrifice but he did not insist on his followers to be vegetarians.

Other food items: Honey, sugar, sugar-cane juice, molasses, and sweet cakes were popular; the spices in common use included salts, ginger, cumin seeds, pepper, turmeric, asafoetida, and vinegar. Commonly used fruits were jujube, mango, rose apple, breadfruit, amalaki, banana, coconut, dates, grapes, parūṣaka, and karamarda.[27] Beverages included juice of mango, jujube, banana, honey, grape, parūṣaka, and sugar-cane juice.

Liquor was manufactured on a large scale and strong wine was sold in shops. Strong liquors were called "madya" but the general varieties widely consumed were classified as "Surā" of five types prepared from rice, flour, and cakes fermented with spices. Maireya was extracted from flowers, fruits, honey, or molasses, and called āsavas. Ariṣta (fermented after decoction) was also available. Vāruṇī – strong liquor – was prepared from madhūka flowers.

This list of food may appear long but it pales before the grand classification of food and drinks in Āyurveda! In one of the longest chapters in his Saṃhitā, Caraka gave a most detailed classification, which grouped food into 10 categories as follows:

1. Śukadhānya (husked grains)
2. Śamīdhānya (pulses)
3. Māṃsa (meats)
4. Śāka (vegetables)
5. Phala (fruits)
6. Harita (greens)
7. Madya (fermented drinks)
8. Jala (waters)
9. Gorasa (milk and milk products)
10. Ikṣu (sugars)

Each category was divided into subgroups with indications of their qualities, effects on doṣas, and other effects on the body. A supplementary list categorised dietary preparations (kṛtānnas) and food additives. A list also provided the names of specific postprandial drinks to be taken after different kinds of meals. The section on "food and drinks" in the Buddhist literature grew into a mighty tree in the Carakasaṃhitā!

Etiquette for dining: We learn that designated posts for supervising the kitchen and common dining rooms existed in Buddhist monasteries.[28] The seating of senior monks and juniors, serving and receiving various items of food, quantities to be served, care in handling food to avoid spilling, picking up and eating spilled food, avoiding too large mouthfuls while eating, putting out the tongue and smacking lips, licking fingers, and many other bits of conduct in the dining room were regulated by rules.[29] These were far more elaborate than the rules indicated by Caraka.[30]

Moderation in eating was strongly urged by Buddhist authorities. Buddhaghosha was of the view that taking only one meal a day will ensure freedom from illness.[31]

Diseases and their treatment

In Buddhist literature diseases are known by several terms including ābādha, āmaya, vyādhi, roga, and ruja, which are familiar to Āyurvedic physicians. Buddhist physicians recognised eight causes for diseases, which were excess of vāta, pitta or kapha, combined excess of the three doṣas, severe or abnormal changes in season, external agencies; effect of karma, and "avoiding dissimilarities (viṣama-hārajāni)."[32] Caraka classified the causes crisply as:

i. Too little or too much use and misuse of senses;
ii. Seasonal upheavals; and
iii. Imprudent conduct (prajñāparādha).

It was also recognised that causes alone could not produce disease and they would have to upset the balance of three doṣas in order to manifest in diseases.

No systematic classification of diseases is seen in Buddhist texts, but Āyurveda offers several classifications. Suśruta mentions a popular and scientific classification that groups diseases as accidental (āgantu), somatic (śārīra), psychic (mānasa), and natural (svābhāvika). He has also described another classification as ādhyatmika (physical), ādhibhautika (caused by physical environment), and ādhidaivika (through acts of nature).

A large number of diseases are mentioned in Buddhist texts; an even larger number are described and classified in Āyurvedic texts under various categories.

Examples of diseases mentioned in Buddhist literature:

- Ajīrṇa (Dyspepsia)
- Atisāra (Diarrhoea)
- Apamāra (Epilepsy)
- Arśa (Piles)
- Udāvarta (Flatulence)
- Unmāda (Insanity)
- Kakṣa (Axillary boil)
- Kaṇdu (Itching)
- Kilāsa (Leucoderma)
- Kukṣiroga (Abdominal disorders – several varieties)
- Kuṣṭa (Leprosy)
- Galagaṇda (Goitre)
- Gharadinnaka (Alcoholism)
- Jvara (Fever)
- Pāṇdu (Jaundice)
- Pakkhaṇdika (Dysentery)
- Pakṣaghāta (Hemiplegia)
- Madhumeha (Diabetes Mellitus)

- Mūrccha (Syncope)
- Lohitapitta (Bleeding disorders)
- Viṣūcikā (Cholera)
- Svāsa (Asthma)
- Sīpada (Elephantiasis)
- Sośa (Pulmonary Tuberculosis)

All these diseases are mentioned in Āyurvedic texts under different classifications and their descriptions systematised under a standard format.

In discussing the treatment of diseases, it would come as no surprise that information is scanty in Buddhist literature because they are not medical but religious texts. As treatment of each disease cannot be satisfactorily discussed, a list of the treatment procedures used in the practice of medicine is given below:

Examples of treatment:

- Dietary regimen (rice gruel)
- Topical application of chunnam, lotus fibres, sulphur
- Ingestion of mud potion (for alcoholism)
- Emesis by giving emetics like madanaphala
- Blood-letting (cupping)
- Specific medications:
    - o ghṛtas (butter, oil, honey, molasses)
    - o Salts (sea salt, rock salt), and
    - o Chunam.

Pañcakarma: Pañcakarma therapy occupies a central place in treating patients in Āyurveda, which employs it to expel excessive and perturbed doṣas from the body. The therapy includes two preparatory procedures – lubricant therapy or oleation (snehana) and body fomentation or sudation (svedana). These are followed by five main procedures – vamana (emesis), virecana (purgation), naśya (nasal purging), kaṣāya-vasti (non-lubricant enema), and sneha-vasti (lubricant enema). Corresponding terms are found in Buddhist texts as follows:

Āyurveda	Buddhist
Vamana	Uddhavirecana
Virecana	Adhovirecana
Naśya	Śiravirecana

There are also descriptions of Buddha undergoing pañcakarma therapy.

Surgical procedures: Surgical procedures are frequently mentioned in Buddhist texts.[33] The term was "Sallakattiya," which corresponds to "Śalyāpahartṛka" of Carakasaṃhitā. Surgery was used for the removal of foreign bodies, cleansing ulcers, excision of anal fistula, removal of dead foetus, and several other conditions. Leech for blood-letting is mentioned in Buddhist literature.[34] Surgical operations for a variety of conditions, surgical training in experimental models, and surgical instruments were described in detail in "Suśrutasaṃhitā."

A few specific conditions treated by surgery are outlined below:

Intussusception (Aṇta-gaṇṭhābādha): The son of a merchant developed intussusception and resultant obstruction of intestine. Jīvaka was permitted by King Bimbisāra to treat the boy.[35] He did a laparotomy, relieved the obstruction, repaired the incision, and patient recovered. Surgery for relieving intestinal obstruction is clearly described in Suśrutasaṃhitā.

Boil (sphoṭa): Incision and drainage of boils and abscesses was often done with a lancet.[36] Sometimes, the healing would be delayed when wound care with sesamum paste/mustard powder/fumigation were done followed by bandaging. Similar accounts are also given in Suśrutasaṃhitā.

Fistula-in-Ano (Bhagandara): Treatment was mainly surgical involving incision, cauterisation, and excision. When a surgeon – Ākāśagotto - operated on the anal fistula of a Bhikku, serious complications made his life miserable and Buddha forbade Bhikkus from undergoing surgery. Detailed techniques for operating on fistula-in-ano are given in Suśrutasaṃhitā (SS). The Kṣārasūtra mentioned briefly in SS is not found in Buddhist literature.

The practice of surgical procedures in Buddhist India, in so far as we observe in available Buddhist texts, makes it clear that surgery was done and had occupied an important place in the over-all management of patient care. Some form of training of surgeons including cadaveric dissection and experimental surgery probably did exist. It is equally clear that these beginnings had blossomed into a calling in Suśruta's time when surgery became "the most important among the branches of Āyurveda because it produces quick results from the use of instruments, alkali, and cautery and comprehends all that the other branches contain. It unbars the gates of heaven and is eternal, virtuous, worthy of high repute, and generous in providing a means for living."[37]

Components of medical treatment: Buddhist texts recognised three key components for carrying out successful treatment of diseases. These were the physician, attendant, and the patient. In Āyurveda, this was expanded to four components by adding drugs and stipulating elaborate credentials for each of the four members. Buddhist Bhikkus had access to hospitals for treatment.[38] The hospital service became more elaborate in Caraka's time.[39]

Vegetable and animal products in treatment: Traditional medicine used vegetable, animal, and mineral products in treating patients. Vegetable products constituted the largest share and was classified in Āyurveda as vanaspati, vīrudha, vānaspatya, and oṣadhi. However, in Buddhist medicine, a classification into five groups was indicated. These are propagated from root (mūlabīja), from stem (khaṇḍabīja), from knot (phaḷubīja), from cutting (aggabīja), and from seed (bījabīja). Each group includes a large number of plants and trees and each has merits in the treatment of various diseases, which are clearly outlined. There are 435 medicinal plants mentioned in the Buddhist writings according Professor Jyotir Mitra.[40] A number of plants mentioned by Caraka are absent in the Buddhist list.

Animal products were used in medical therapy in Buddhist India. Examples are milk and milk products, animal fat, and cow's urine. Caraka and Suśruta recommend many more but animal products are a small part of Āyurvedic formulary, which was dominated by vegetables.

Among metals and minerals, Buddhist literature does not mention the use of any kind of metal in medical treatment, though they do classify loha – metals - into four kinds.[41] Caraka describes gold, the odure of metals, five baser metals (silver, copper, lead, tin, iron), sand, lime, and minerals such as read arsenic, gems, salts, red chalk, and antimony as drugs of earthly origin (bhauma).[42] Mercury was not mentioned. Metals and minerals were only a tiny part of Āyurvedic formulary. Rasaśāstra appeared centuries after Caraka and Suśruta.

Buddhist India through the eyes of a Chinese pilgrim

Hieun-Tsiang – the distinguished Chinese scholar and pilgrim – spent several years in India in the fifth century CE. Buddhism was already in decline and travel in India difficult but his observant eye missed nothing. He found that physicians treated patients mostly by dietary regime and medical decoctions; hospitals provided free service in cities to poor patients. At the age of seven, children were instructed in five vidyas which included sabdavidya, śilpa vidya, cikitsa vidya, hetu vidya, and adhyātma vidya. Cikitsa included secret charms, medicinal gems, acupuncture, and mugwort. It is uncertain whether acupuncture refers to a little-known procedure which Suśruta refers to. This was making a tiny incision near a marma far away from the seat of the disease and the cut producing a beneficial effect on the distantly located disease. Mugwort is Rauwolfia serpentina which is not mentioned in Bṛhattrayī. Hieun Tsiang also saw a hall built by Jīvaka for the Buddha to give sermons in Rajgir and the residence of Jīvaka nearby - both in ruins. He commented, "sick people fast for seven days, when most get well. Thereafter, they consult physicians who give medications." He had much praise for Nāgārjuna and his achievements in alchemy which had taken roots in India.

Spread of Āyurvedic ideas through Buddhist channels

Āyurveda is practiced all over India with regional variations. On the other hand, Āyurvedic ideas like tridoṣa, pathya, pañcakarma, and herbal therapy have travelled not only across India but also beyond to Sri Lanka, Nepal, Tibet, Central Asia, and East Asia. The Chinese pilgrims Fa-Hien, and Hieun-Tsiang spread these ideas in China in the fourth and fifth centuries CE, not to replace traditional Chinese medicine but to widen their cultural horizon. This vast spread of ideas was powered by the Buddhist current which accepted everyone with open arms regardless of caste, language, beliefs, customs, and geography. Wherever Buddhism went, Āyurveda joined as a companion because it was an integral part of the Buddhist code for living. Buddhist scholars and physicians taught Sanskrit barring no one and opened the treasure house of new medical learning to people wherever they lived. At the same time, regional languages were freely used in learning and local practices in therapy of proven efficacy adopted into mainstream Āyurveda. The reputed practice of "pizhichil," "dhāra," etc. in Kerala are prime examples of this liberal culture of adoption and assimilation which carried Āyurvedic ideas to faraway places in Central Asia. The Bower manuscript is a vivid illustration of this disseminative phenomenon. Col Bower, stationed in India, went on a punitive expedition to Kucha in Central Asia and came upon a monastery in ruins and a manuscript therein. Having accomplished his mission, he returned to India with the manuscript and gifted it to the Royal Asiatic Society in Calcutta. Dr Hoernle, a great scholar, recognised the historical importance of the manuscript of Buddhist authorship. It was an ancient Āyurvedic treatise in Sanskrit written in Brahmi script with many extracts from Bhela Saṃhitā and references to Suśruta; but none to Caraka. The historical importance of the "Bower manuscript" lies in the fact that it is one of the few, if not the only, Āyurvedic text available which was composed before Carakasaṃhitā when Buddhist physicians were the leaders of Āyurveda. Though Āyurveda was transformed by the trinity of Caraka, Suśruta, and Vāgbhaṭa, the Buddhist ring is clearly audible in the practice of Āyurveda even today.

Learned assemblies

Learned Assemblies - pariṣad – were often held by monks to discuss disputed questions. The Anguttara Nikāya mentions 10 types of assemblies covering social, ethical, philosophical, and other domains.[43] Buddha divided the first assembly into two kinds; those focussed on frivolous or trivial issues characterised by sound and fury (uttānā), and those dealing with serious issues marked by mature and thoughtful discussions (gambhīra). There were also other classifications which indicate the importance attached to intellectual debates on all subjects of importance. These assemblies had great appeal to all educated Indians and their echo can be heard in Carakasaṃhitā which again divides assemblies as those of the wise (jnānavatīpariṣad), those of fools (mūdhapariṣad), those of friendly or hostile participants, etc. In a long chapter, Caraka gives a detailed description of debates, the logical parameters of debates and the techniques to win debates. This was important for physicians who wished to establish the authority of their doctrines, to refute false views, and win recognition from the King. The logical content of Caraka's discussion was so pioneering that Professor Dasgupta held that many of his definitions and postulates antedated Nyāya Sūtra.

References:

1. S N Dasgupta. "*A History of Indian philosophy,*" Vol 1: PP2. Motilal Banarasidas. Delhi 1997.
2. T W Rhys Davids. *Buddhist India* Page 2 – 3. Low Price Publications. Delhi 2010.
3. *DN* 2. 27
4. *CS* Sūtra: 30: 28
5. *DN* 1: 215
6. *MN* iii: 115
7. *SN* XXXVI. II: 3.21
8. *MP* IV: 62 1 bid J. II, 191 (two references)
9. *AN* VII: 7.9
10. *VM,* VIII: 25
11. *AN* III: 7
12. *AN* VI: 3.9
13. *DP* XV: 8
14. *VP,* Parivāra VII. 3.13
15. *VP,* Parājika I. 2.70, *MP,* JJ, 30 *CS* 15:72
16. *VP,* CV, V: 15.40 *CS,* I: 5.72
17. *MP,* II. 17
18. *J,* 1: 31

19. *VP*, Pac, VII: 75. 231
20. *VM*, I, 81
21. *SS*, IV: 24.30
22. *VP*, CV. X: 19.35
23. *CS Sūtra*, V: 93-94
24. *DN*, 30 (Lakkana sutta)
25. *AN*, III: 250
26. *VP*, Pāraj IV: 5. 50
27. *J*, II: 260, 547; 537
28. *VP*, Pārāj: 1.2.119
29. *VP*, Pāc. VII. 31-92
30. *CS* Vimana: 1.24
31. *VM*, II. 38
32. *MP*, IV: 63
33. *DN*, 1.2.27
34. *MP*, VII. 5.19
35. *VP*, *MV*: VIII. 5.8
36. *VP*, *MV*: VI 2.8
37. *SS* Sūtra, 1: 14 - 21
38. *SN*, IV. 210
39. *CS* Sūtras, 15: 5 – 7
40. Jyotir Mitra, *Āyurvedic Material in Buddhist literature*, Jyotiralok Prakashan, Varanasi. 1985. Page 205.
41. *Jyotir Mitra* 1bid. Page 210.
42. *CS Sūtra* I: 70
43. *AN* II, 5: 1 - 10

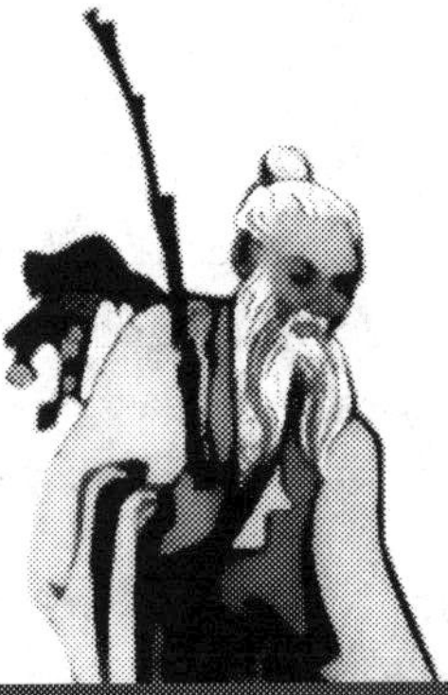

CHAPTER 3

Evolution of Āyurveda from Caraka to Vāgbhaṭa

From Caraka to Vāgbhaṭa - Historical Pointers:

Caraka is believed to have lived in the Punjab–Kashmir region during the reign of Kāniṣka in the famous Kuṣāna Empire. There are dissenting views on his name and location, a claim is that his name merely implies his affiliation to an itinerant class of physicians, and that he was Patañjali who composed the Mahābhāṣya in the second century BCE. The majority of scholars favour the Kuṣāna empire view and point to a Chinese text quoted by Professor Sylvain Levi, which claimed that Kāniṣka had two favourite companions in his court – Aśvaghoṣa – the poet and author of Buddhacarita and Caraka – the physician.[1] Caraka immortalised himself by redacting Agniveśatantra – a text in Āyurveda which had been acclaimed for centuries earlier. Carakasaṃhitā continues to remain the foundational text of Āyurveda even today as it deals with life in its entirety and in conformity with the definition of Āyurveda. Apart from health and disease and how to remain well and escape from illness, its vast province includes philosophical themes in epistemology, bioethics, and logical parameters of debate, training of ideal physicians, environmental protection, and a host of other ideas which enliven the central theme of the practice of medicine. No wonder his text was translated into Persian and European languages and a medical club was founded in his name in New York in the 19th century by eminent physicians, including Sir William Osler. The Carakasaṃhitā was lost in parts over many centuries and was restored and revised by a Kashmiri physician Dṛḍhabala in the fourth century CE.

The second authoritative text after Caraka's among the "Great Three" (Bṛhattrayī) of Āyurveda bears the name of Suśruta, who is believed to have lived in Banaras before the Buddha. His teacher was a King of Kaśi – Divodasa, who was so great a physician that he was regarded as a descendant of Lord Dhanvantari. Hoernlé who was a pioneer of Indic studies in the early 20th century held the view that the original Suśruta Tantra, which had probably been redacted more than once "admittedly belongs to a much earlier period, possibly as early as 1000 BC." Hessler had advanced this view earlier in his Latin edition of Suśrutasaṃhitā. Another clear pointer to Suśruta's date is the reference to him by Pāṇini who used his name as a familiar example in his sūtras.[2] As Pāṇini lived around 500 BCE in Takṣaśilā and Banaras was thousands of miles away, Suśruta would have lived much earlier for Pāṇini to use Suśruta's name as a familiar example. An additional and important evidence for Suśruta's antiquity is that he makes no reference to trephining of the skull among the many procedures he described, whereas Jīvaka's life recorded in the Jātakas has detailed references to the dramatic success of this operation done by him on a merchant with the permission of King Bimbisāra. Jīvaka was the physician of King Bimbisāra and Lord Buddha and his trephining operation did not obviously exist in Suśruta's period. Suśruta's original treatise was lost and there is general agreement that Nāgārjuna redacted the Suśrutasaṃhitā in the current form in the fourth century CE. The "Saṃhitās of Caraka and Suśruta" became the eternal favourites ever since and continue to be used by physicians, botanists, pharmacologists, scholars, sociologists, and historians. They are taught to tens of thousands of students of Āyurveda every year.

In the sixth century CE, Sindhudeśa (Sind) gave birth to a physician - extraordinary and gifted poet Vāgbhaṭa, whose name is associated with two texts, which became classics. These are the Aṣṭāṅgasaṅgraha (AS) and the Aṣṭāṅgahṛdaya (AH), which are both authoritative texts. There is however no agreement among scholars whether these were composed by the same Vāgbhaṭa or whether AS was written by Vāgbhaṭa Senior and AH by Vāgbhaṭa Junior. What is beyond doubt is that AH clearly states that it is a distillate of AS and is written to suit the changing times (yagānurūpa) in "neither too short nor too long" a format for the students and practitioners. It is also clear that Vāgbhaṭa was a devotee of Lord Buddha and his authority as a physician was matched by his poetic excellence. He pointed out that mere antiquity did not confer greatness or authority on medical texts and drew attention to the fact that while generations continued to study Caraka and Suśruta for centuries, but not Bhela who was no less ancient and was a fellow student of Agniveśa whose text Caraka had redacted.[3] What really matters is the intrinsic merit and authority of a text, which should equal those of the authoritative texts of the distant past. He was supremely confident that his AH was the ambrosia emerging from the churning of the Ayurvedic Ocean.

Diseases in India; a Count from CS: What was the pattern of diseases among the population in North-West India in the first century when Caraka redacted his encyclopaedic Saṃhitā? This is a question of importance in the history of medicine, sociology, and epidemiology which deals with the prevalence and spread of diseases in communities. As epidemiological studies were non-existent anywhere in the world 2000 years ago, it is possible only to study the descriptions of diseases in CS and make a rough estimate of the prevalence of diseases in the Caraka's period. This is based on the observations that a textbook of general medicine meant for students and practitioners would pay greater attention and devote more pages to diseases prevalent at that particular time because that would provide the most relevant information to the medical profession. An edition of the same text book published 60 years later would have different priorities as the prevalence of diseases would have changed in the community and the number of references in the text would change in response to the prevailing disease load. A look at the emphasis given to say, typhoid fever and "coronary thrombosis" in a textbook of general medicine published in the first decade of the 20th century would show many more references to typhoid fever than to coronary thrombosis; in contrast, an edition of the same text published in the last quarter of the 20th century would have far fewer references to typhoid than to coronary thrombosis, thanks to the epidemiological transition in the community, which implies a decline of infectious diseases and the rise of non-communicable diseases. This is in line with improved living conditions and socio-economic progress. A study was in fact, carried out to count the references to a group of infectious and non-communicable diseases in a digitised version of CS, which was provided by Professor Yamashita of the Kyoto University.[4] Larger the number of references, the more common would be the disease and, conversely, fewer the references, less common would they be. The search in what could be called archeo-epidemiology yielded 883 references to infectious diseases and conditions: fevers (jvara) 430, tuberculosis (śoṣa) 130, sores and ulcers (vraṇa) 87, digestive disorders (ajīrṇa) 84, skin disease including leprosy (kuṣṭha) 64, cellulitis (visarpa) 55, cholera (viṣūcikā) 22, and abscesses (vidradhi) 11. Against these counts, non-infectious conditions had a total count of 581: gaseous lumps of the abdomen (gulma) 132, gastrointestinal bleeding (raktapitta) 95, piles (arśa) 77, epilepsy (apasmāra) 61, heart disease (hṛdroga) 59, diabetes (prameha) 51, diseases of pallor (pāṇḍuroga) 49, insanity (unmāda) 35, and alcoholic disorders (madātyaya) 22. These figures clearly suggest that infectious diseases were far more common and constituted a far greater disease load on the community in Caraka's India. This exercise also tells us that small pox (masūrika) was virtually unknown then as it had only two doubtful references. Similarly, severe malnutrition and cachexia were not observed in the study.

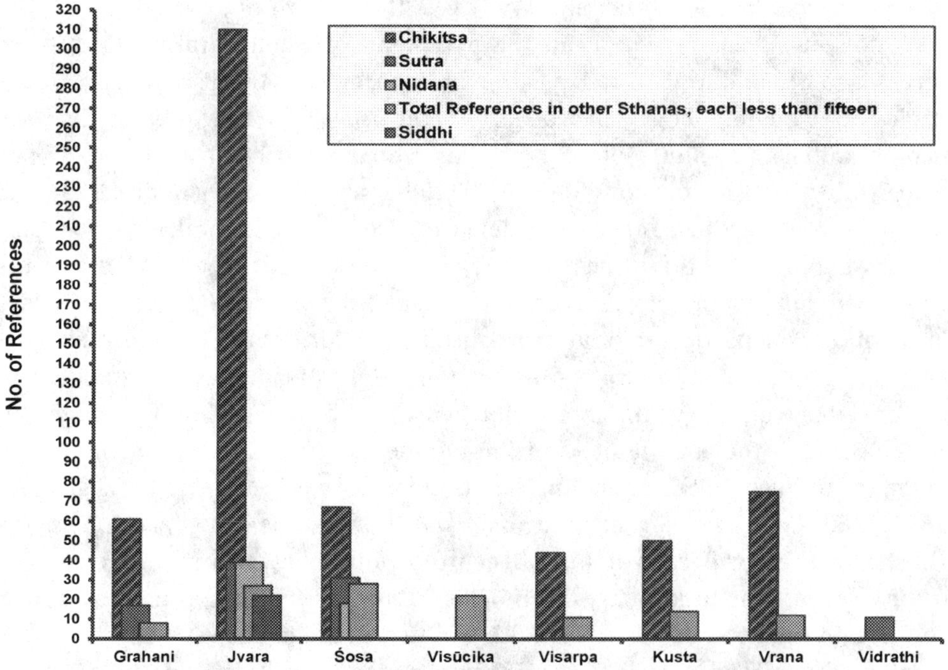

Fig. 1: References to infectious diseases and infected conditions

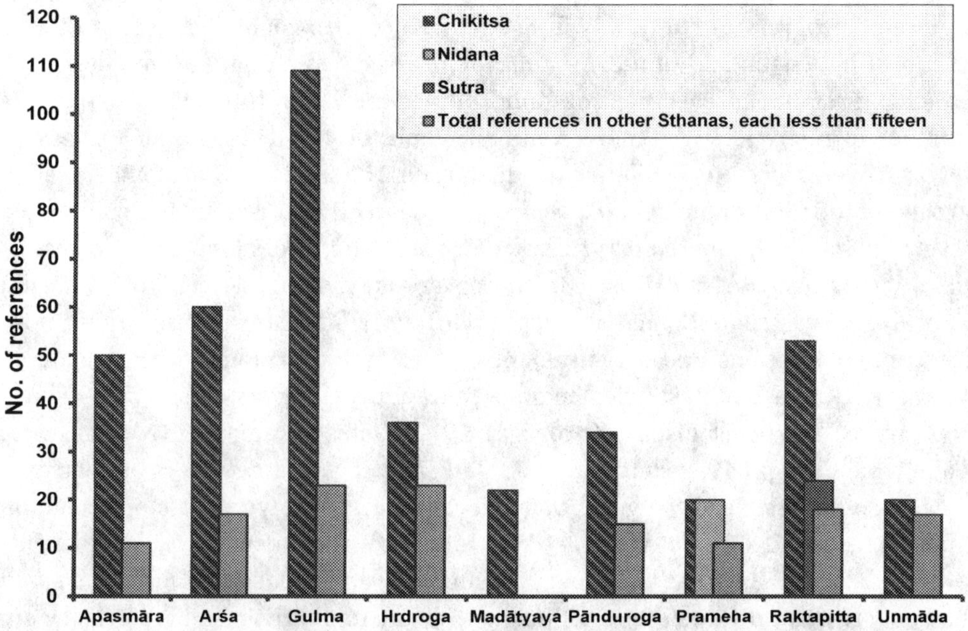

Fig. 2: References to non-infectious diseases

Trends in the Practice of Medicine from Caraka to Vāgbhaṭa: The five centuries from Caraka to Vāgbhaṭa were arguably the "golden period" in the history of Āyurveda. It witnessed the redaction of the "Saṃhitās of Caraka and Suśruta," the composition of "Aṣṭāṅgasaṅgraha and Aṣṭāṅgahṛdaya" by Vāgbhaṭa, a flourishing network of Gurukulas, spread of Āyurveda all over India and abroad, translations of Bṛhattrayī into Persian, Tibetan, and other languages, and the systematization of the study and practice of Āyurveda as we know it today. It would be interesting to know the trends if any, in the practice of Āyurveda during these centuries even if the historical information is incomplete in the ancient texts. Were the basic doctrines, diagnosis and treatment of diseases, and medical procedures, which were followed in the period of Caraka practiced without change in the time of Vāgbhaṭa? If there were changes, did they indicate any trends? What was the status of the Dhanvantari tradition of surgery during these five centuries?

A comparative study of the practice of Āyurveda in the period of Caraka and Vāgbhaṭa was therefore carried out with reference to doctrines and philosophical ideas, treatment of diseases, and medical procedures.[5] The examples chosen for the study were doctrines, tuberculosis, and pañcakarma. The findings of the comparative study can be summarised as follows:

Doctrines and Philosophical Ideas: The doctrine of the cosmos as a macrocosm and man as a microcosm was central in Caraka's philosophy. The homology of the five elements (pañcabhūta), which constitute the cosmos and the human body, played an important role in his approach to the choice of drugs and diet for patients. Similarly, Caraka paid great attention to guṇas taken from "vaiśeṣika" in understanding substances (dravyas), which underlie food and drugs. He described the logical parameters of debate for physicians so elaborately that Professor Dasgupta claimed that "Nyāyasūtra" had borrowed some of these ideas from Caraka! Lastly, Caraka pioneered the original sāṅkhya doctrine of 24 "tatvas" in the process of evolution (pariṇāma). All these profound doctrines received decreasing attention in AS and AH. Medicine had become more of a practical art in five centuries with less emphasis on philosophy. One should look less for the abstract and the profound and more for the concrete in AS and AH, which were written for the busy practitioners and young trainees. The ritual for the initiation of trainees and the grand oath to be administered by the Acharya to the student, which were fully described by Caraka received scant attention in AH, which could even suggest a decline of the Gurukula tradition.

Treatment of Diseases: When we turn to the treatment of diseases and look at the dreaded disease of tuberculosis, the above study showed that the clinical picture of the disease, prognosis, diagnostic criteria, the bearing of the physical condition of the patient on the choice of treatment, and the role of medical procedures had changed little between the dates of CS, AS and AH. The significant changes were limited to the modifications, additions, and deletions in the formulations used by physicians in treating patients.

Medical Procedures: Regarding medical procedures, enemas stood out in the time zones of Caraka and Vāgbhaṭa in terms of the universality of their applications, acclaimed efficacy in treating diseases and maintaining good health. The rationale for their use, classifications of complications and other practical details received great attention in CS, AS and AH. The changes were limited to the reduction in the number of formulations used for enema and the elimination of peripheral topics such as enema for quadrupeds.

It is significant that no major advances at the doctrinal or practical levels had occurred in the long period between the redaction of CS and the composition of AS and AH. The observations of the Chinese pilgrim Hiuen Tsiang in the sixth century had indicated the general decline of Buddhist places of worship and institutions of learning in India. Most alarming was the eclipse of Suśruta's legacy during this period as surgical procedures disappeared from the mainstream of Āyurveda and survived precariously in the hands of illiterate people in the fringes of the society. This was a huge set back to Āyurveda.

Much has been written in history on the powerful Gupta Empire, which had given liberal support for two centuries to learned professions and religion throughout their vast territories. The eclipse of the Gupta empire coincided with a decline on every front in India – political, military, trade, and cultural – in the sixth century CE. The effect of the demise of the Gupta Empire on the set back to Āyurveda still remains to be investigated.

Āyurveda after Vāgbhaṭa: Āyurveda faced a long phase of almost a 1000 years of stagnation after Vāgbhaṭa. All the intellectual and educational activities declined during this long period when Āyurveda ceased to have great centres of learning, and the Gurukula system declined beyond any hope of recovery. The period of stagnation was however not a "dark age" of intellectual stupor. Three important texts – "Laghutrayī", named after Śārṅgadhara, Mādhava, and Bhāva Miśra appeared, which broke new ground. While Sāraṇgadhara mentioned "pulse" in medical diagnosis for the first time, Mādhava devoted his entire book to the diagnostic process, which was innovative. Bhāva Misra recorded syphilis for the first time as his book appeared after the entry of Portuguese in India.

Another development of importance was the growth of Rasaśāstra which had its origin in Arab medicine. The classics of Bṛhattrayī had hardly mentioned mercury and their references to metal derived products and minerals constituted no more than a tiny part of the Ayurvedic formulary. The encounter with Arab medicine which used mercury, metal derived products and minerals extensively was followed by an explosive interest among Ayurvedic physicians in alchemy which had centres in Nalanda, Vikramaśila, Udāntapura, and Śriśailam. Alchemy was practised by men of all castes except Brahmins. While European alchemists were on the trail of the philosopher's stone, the Siddhas in India gave a religious spin to alchemy as a form of Tantra and as a means to self-realisation. The Siddha endeavour focussed on developing a power which, on transfer to mercury, would empower mercury to convert base metals to gold. Side by side, they also made efforts to empower mercury to convert old body cells into young ones. These two attainments were termed Loha Siddhi and Deha Siddhi which were eagerly sought and zealously guarded as a secret. Nāgārjuna was a pioneer of alchemy who had passed away when Hiuen Tsiang visited his birth place and heaped praise on him. A later visitor in eigth century CE was Al Beruni who too acclaimed Nāgārjuna's work. P C Ray traced the development of chemistry in India to alchemy after detailed studies including the editing and publication of ancient texts such as "Rasārṇava."

While the examples cited above indicate that progress had not ended after Vāgbhaṭa, it was equally clear that heavy clouds had gathered in the Ayurvedic firmament. This was partly due to political reasons because the Muslim rulers in India preferred Unani to the detriment of Āyurveda and also, because the social fabric in India was torn up so perversely that large sections of people who used their hands to make a living including surgeons, craftsmen, weavers, medical assistants, and many others found themselves classed as "low caste" and denied the benefits of education and social mobility. Cadaveric dissection and experimental surgery in pumpkin, leather, jackfruit and so on to learn surgical techniques disappeared from the training of physicians; admirable procedures described by Suśruta including the plastic reconstruction of the nose and ear, removal of bladder stone, couching for cataract and reduction of fractures bid good bye to the mainstream of Āyurveda. Vaidyas no longer cared to perform any of these procedures. We have eye witness accounts[6,7] by qualified observers during the 19th century CE who watched illiterate and "low caste" men doing skilled operations such as plastic reconstruction of the nose in Pune and couching for cataract in Coimbatore. The operators had learnt the technique from an earlier generation but had no understanding of anatomy or the rationale for the sequential steps of the procedure being done. To every question why is this step being taken? Why not make it easier by another method, the practitioner's answer was always "I don't know, my father taught me to do it this way, which is perfect." This was identical to the response of bone setters, dayis and many others who provided much needed service to the society. It was as if their brain had been uncoupled from their hand! It was this grim picture which made P C Ray observe:

> The arts thus being relegated to the lower castes, and the professions made hereditary, a certain degree of fineness, delicacy, and deftness in manipulation was no doubt achieved, but this was accomplished at a terrible cost. The intellectual portion of the community being thus withdrawn from active participation in arts, the how and why of a phenomenon – the coordination of cause and effect were lost sight of. The spirit of inquiry gradually died out among a nation, naturally prone to speculation and metaphysical subtleties, and India for once bade adieu to experimental and inductive sciences. Her soil was made morally unfit for the birth of a Boyle, a Descartes, or a Newton, and her very name was all but expunged from the map of the scientific world for a time.[8]

These were the cruel circumstances which Āyurveda faced in the 18th and 19th centuries CE, when British rule established itself in India. British scientists took the initiative in setting up institutions for modern science and medical education in India in the 19th century CE and they took special interest in the study of medicinal plants. Roxburgh, for example, was a pioneer in documenting the botanical wealth of Bengal and was admired by J C Bose. However, they regarded Āyurveda as no more than traditional "herbal therapy" devoid of science and refused to promote its study or practice. While the Government of British India established over 10 research institutions all over India in the late 19th and early 20th century such as, Central Research Institute, Kasauli, School of Tropical Medicine, Kolkata, Plague Research Institute, Mumbai, Nutritional Research Laboratory, Coonoor, and King Institute, Guindy, Āyurveda found no place in the promotional agenda. Early 20th century was the worst of times for Āyurveda, when it enjoyed little support from the State, the profession of Vaidyas was demoralised and crippled, Gurukula system for training young physicians had collapsed, and the rulers and western educated Indians looked down upon traditional Indian medicine as mere mumbo jumbo. The spirit of Āyurveda was kept alive in this dark hour by pioneers here and there in the country notably, Gananath Sen in Kolkata, Lakshmipathy in Chennai, P S Varier in Kottakkal, and a few other heroes.

References:

1. J A Soc Nat. *Notes Sur les Indo-Scythes*, December 1896. Page 451, 473.
2. *Aṣṭādhyāyi* IV: 3.107: 1 bid VI: 2.37: 1 bid II: 1: 60

3. Uttara. *AH*. 40: 84-89
4. M S Valiathan, *The Legacy of Caraka*. Orient Blackswan, Hyderabad. 2003. Page XXIV–XIVII.
5. M S Valiathan, *The Legacy of Vāgbhaṭa*, Orient Blackswan, Hyderabad. 2009. Introduction, Page XV–XVIII.
6. H Scott Bombay, India Office Library London. Personal Communication. Dharampal.
7. *Jaggi O P Medicine in India: Modern period*, Ed D P Chattopadhyaya OUP Delhi (2000). Page 234.
8. P C Ray (1956). *History of Chemistry in Ancient and Medieval India*. Indian Chemistry Society, Kolkata Page 248.

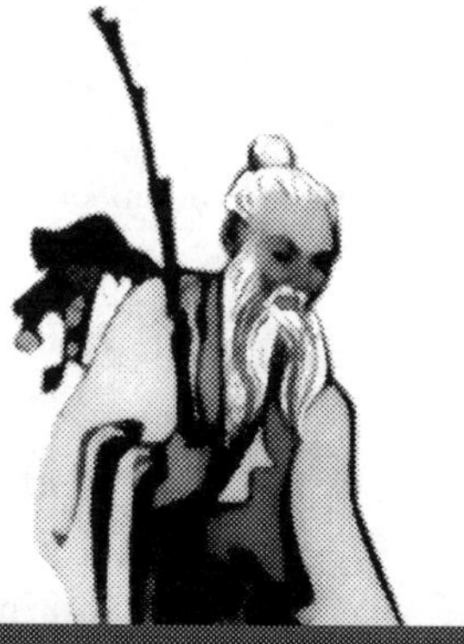

CHAPTER 4

Philosophical Ideas in Āyurveda

Why should a good and successful Āyurvedic physician care to know anything about philosophy? He need not have knowledge of philosophical systems like metaphysics, epistemology, aesthetics, or politics to practice medicine. Of all the branches of philosophy, only ethics in so far as it urges one to do what is right is of relevance to the practicing physicians. While ethics dominates the oath of the initiate in Carakasamhita (CS), the bulk of philosophical discourse does not help the physician to become more efficient, rich or famous, or teach him how to make friends and influence people. Yet, Caraka was notably inclined to philosophy and excelled as a philosopher–physician. It was characteristic of him to add a significant line at the end of a long classification of 600 drugs with numerous formulations and ingredients, "while this would suffice for the practice of the average physician of low intelligence, it would also push the frontiers of knowledge for the thoughtful and wise."[1] His philosophical inquiries and allusions were addressed to the "thoughtful and wise" among physicians who had the gift of curiosity to know the meaning of life on earth, "happiness and unhappiness, wholesomeness and unwholesomeness," the world in which we find ourselves and how our life ought to be lived.[2] In short, Caraka added a touch of the "soul's adventures in the cosmos" to the science and art of medicine. Therein lies the fountain-head of philosophical ideas, which enliven Āyurveda.

Individual and the cosmos; pañcabhūta as common substratum

Pañcabhūta or five elements is a basic philosophical doctrine of Āyurveda. The physical world is known to us through our five senses – sight, hearing, smell, taste, and touch, which are located in our eye, ear, nose, tongue, and skin. As properties are not independent entities and must reside within substances, there must be five elements (bhūtas), which correspond to the five sensations. These elements are not perceived in their pure state because our daily experience of substances suggests that they consist of the five elements in a mixed form. Each bhūta is marked by a specific quality; ether (ākāśa) by sound, air (vāyu) by touch, fire (agni) by light, water (ap) by taste, and earth (pṛthvī) by smell. It must also be noted that bhūtas increase progressively in density as they range from ether to earth; secondly, each succeeding bhūta in the series possesses not only its own characteristic property but also the property of its predecessors in the series. All the substances, which constitute the physical world including our food, drinks, medications, and body consists of the five bhūtas. The homology of the five elements in the food we consume, our body and the world around us has profound implications in our life and the practice of medicine. Diseases are manifestations of a disturbed equilibrium marked by perturbations in the level of body constituents (dhātus). These perturbations may be due to increase or decrease, which need to be restored to normal levels by giving drugs or food with properties opposed to those of the perturbed constituents. This is a basic method in therapeutics, which is hardly possible unless the body constituents and administered substances are homologous in their composition.[3]

The pañcabhūta doctrine is no more than a part of a grander concept which unites the individual and the cosmos in a continuum.[4] Whatever exists in the cosmos exists in the individual and, in the reverse, whatever exists in the individual is found in the universe. These constituents are countless but, at the most basic level; six cosmic constituents can be identified, which have their indicators in the body. These are the five bhūtas and the formless Brahman, whose indicators in the body are listed by Caraka.[5] Indeed, the identification of the individual with the cosmos and, conversely, that of cosmos with the individual, was regarded as the true measure of knowledge. This discovery would open the royal pathway to the end of sorrow and everlasting bliss.[6]

Categories of all that exists (Vaiśeṣika)

According to Professor Dasgupta, "The whole foundation of his (Caraka's) medical physics is based on vaiśeṣika physics."[7] This may look surprising to a physician unless he remembers Caraka's universal definition of Āyurveda as the "measure of life happy and unhappy and wholesome and unwholesome."[8] For Caraka, man as a microcosm and cosmos as a macrocosm, interchanging and interacting perpetually, was an article of faith. It was impossible for him to view the administration of a remedy to treat an illness without being conscious that the substances constituting the remedy were homologous to the perturbed constituents of the patient's body and, at the same time, opposed to the properties of the perturbed constituents. It was natural for him to concern himself with the categorisation of all that exists, which had been the preoccupation of vaiśeṣika philosophers even prior to him.

Unlike Vedanta which negated all other than Brahman as "midhyā," vaiśeṣika was a pluralistic system which did not dismiss patent facts of experience but admitted that at the root of every perception these must be something to which the perception was due. Accordingly, vaiśeṣika classified all precepts and concepts (padārthas) of experience into six categories, which Caraka adopted.[9] However, his adoption was qualified and partial because he took only what was necessary for him to build a rational basis for therapeutics (yuktivyapāśraya). Consider guṇas – a category mentioned in the Vaiśeṣikasūtra of Kaṇāda. While the original Sūtra mentioned 40 guṇas under sensations and physical, mental, and intellectual groups, Caraka focused attention only on 20 physical properties such as heavy/light and hot/cold, which are important from a physician's point of view. Sometimes, he adopted terms from Vaiśeṣikasūtra only to give them a different meaning. For example; parā and aparā, are abstract terms used in vaiśeṣika with reference to intellectual functions, but they are used by Caraka to indicate the superior and inferior qualities of locale, climate, etc., in relation to health. Similarly, sāmānya and viśeṣa, which are class concepts in vaiśeṣika are applied to members of a group with similar and dissimilar properties by Caraka (Table 1). Caraka was a master builder, who had expert knowledge of building materials from different quarries and picked what he needed from wherever they were located and crafted them to raise the edifice of medicine.

Table 1:

Term	Vaiśeṣika	Caraka
Para/ Apara	Indicate remote/near in time and space	Superior/Inferior in reference to geography, season, etc. e.g.: A dry country is para (superior); a moist, humid country is apara (inferior)
Samyōga/ Vibhāga	Union of things, which were separate/separation of things, which were in union	Mixing up two or more substances/ their separation
Sāmānya/ Viśeṣa	A certain property resides in many things and is shared/ when the property is regarded as distinguishing them from other things	When a like substance is added to another like substance they increase the bulk/when unlike substance is added, the bulk reduces

Means of accessing knowledge

The origins and sources of knowledge were of great interest to nyāya, vaiśeṣika, sāṅkhya, Buddhist, and Jaina philosophers. While vaiśeṣika and Buddhists accepted only perception (pratyakṣa) and inference (anumāna) as sources, sāṅkhya added śabda (testimony) as a valid source: nyāya added a fourth, upamāna (analogy). This fourfold division of knowledge also admits that the manner of the manifestation of knowledge would be different in each case. Thus, inference and śabda are different sources (pramāṇas) though they may point to the same object indicated by perception.[10]

According the Caraka, the sources of knowledge are testimony (śabda), perception, inference, and reasoning (yukti). As always, his approach to philosophical themes reflected the credo of a physician.

Testimony: A physician is obliged to obtain knowledge from wise persons (āpta) lest he should be condemned to repeat earlier mistakes committed in medical practice. But the āptas "authority" is not limited to knowledge. He should be free from rajas and tamas, and be austere, disciplined, and wise. His knowledge should span the past, present, and future. Incapable of lying, his words should leave no room for ambiguity.[11] Scriptural revelation could also be regarded as "śabda" provided it does not contradict reason. Śabda covers all aspects of the causation, specific features, signs and symptoms, treatment, complications, and prognosis of diseases.[12]

Perception: Perception by senses arises from the contact of sense organs with objects and involves the senses (indriyas), their specific objects (arthas), contact of senses with objects (sannikarṣa), and cognition of the contact (jnāna). The cognitive process involves the mind (manas), which couples the cognitive product with the self. Though perception is handicapped by diverse factors such as the minuteness of the object, too much distance, infirmity of sense organs, and mental instability, it plays a vital role in medical diagnosis. Except for the sense of taste, all senses of the physician contribute to the examination of the patient. Taste alone is examined indirectly by, for example, watching flies approaching a diabetic or vomited blood being shunned by crows and dogs.[13]

Inference: Inference begins where perception stops, but it is always preceded by perception. Inference has three types and three tenses: the consequent from the precedent, the precedent from the consequent, and one member of a pair of complementarities from each other. Physicians use inferences of all types, which are used extensively in making a diagnosis and assessing the efficacy of treatment. To give examples, for the pair of complementarities, fear from anxious expression; for precedent from the consequent, sexual intercourse from pregnancy; for consequent from the precedent, fruit from the seed. In Āyurveda, inference also covers comparison (upamāna) and an example is the view that the growth of the foetus from six dhātus is analogous to the growth of crops from a combination of water, planting, seed, and climate.

Reason: Caraka[14] assigned an independent status to reason among the means of increasing knowledge while other authorities included it in "inference." However, his concept of reason involves a series of thought processes. For example, it is not possible to predict a good or poor harvest from the quality of the seed alone: it would be necessary to know other factors such as the quality of soil, amount of rainfall, manure, and so on. Only on a full consideration of all the concerned factors one could make an informed forecast of a good or poor harvest.

Logical parameters of debate

In the Nyāyasūtra, disputes are classified into vāda, jalpa, and vitaṇda. Vāda is an informed discussion to ascertain truth, jalpa aims to demolish the adversary's point of view rightly or wrongly, and vitaṇda merely picks holes in the opponent's case without advancing one's own arguments. These disputations among peers were highly esteemed by physicians as a means to establish the diagnosis of a disease in a patient or the choice of a particular line of treatment; they were equally welcomed as a forum for a physician to present his doctrine or therapeutic innovation for a debate among peers for approval. The art of winning a debate was so highly prized that Caraka devoted an entire chapter "roga-bhiṣag-jitīyam"[15] to a discussion on the logical parameters of holding a debate. Caraka discussed in detail friendly and hostile assemblies where one may have to defend his doctrine or views and how one's strategy had to be tailored to suit the intellectual calibre and mentality of the audience.

In this kind of debate, mastery of one's subject alone was no guarantee of victory; one had to understand the abilities and vulnerabilities of the opponent and have the presence of mind to evaluate one's own strength vis-à-vis that of the opponent. The attitude, competence, and impartiality of the assembly also had to be kept in mind. Caraka recommended many tactics to win the debate but cautioned that anger and bad temper have no place in a noble assembly. He insisted that a physician discussant should be familiar with the technical terms touching upon debates. He listed 44 terms and covered in full every scientific aspect of debate.[16] He concluded by arguing that debates among physicians should be confined to the topics in Āyurveda and not a word should be spoken which was not well thought out and which was out of place or lacking in scriptural authority. Whatever is said should be backed by reason because debates based on reason are free from ill feeling, and they advance the objectives of medicine by sharpening the intellect.

Dasgupta points out that no work earlier than Caraka's in Hindu, Buddhist, or Jain literature treats logical subjects including inference and parameters of debate found in the CS.[17] But the absence of terms such as pūrvavat and śeṣavat in relation to inference in Caraka and their presence in Nyāyasūtra would suggest a process of subsequent refinement of nomenclature after CS was composed. This trend is equally true in regard to Caraka's definition of perception as a combined operation of sense object, sense, mind and soul, and its more elaborate treatment in Nyāyasūtra. Both these examples would clearly suggest that the logical parameters of debate in CS antedated Nyāyasūtra of Akṣapāda.

Evolution of the cosmos

An individual represents a union of five elements (pañcabhūtas) and consciousness (cetana). At a subtler level, the individual is comprised of 24 constituents (caturvimśati-tatva), which are the mind, 10 sense organs, five sense objects, and eight components of nature. These eight components of nature in turn are sequentially avyakta, mahat, ahaṅkāra, and five bhūtas.[18] Caraka makes no references to "tanmātra" as the forerunners of bhūtas.

The evolution of the 24 constituents which comprise the individual had been a major subject of debate among India's philosophical systems especially sāṅkhya. The doctrine of the evolution of prakṛti occupies a central position in the sāṅkhya system of philosophy. The sāṅkhya doctrine of evolution based on 24 constituents did itself evolve in later centuries as a doctrine based on 25 constituents (pañcavimśati). According to the original sāṅkhya doctrine of 24 constituents, attributed to Caraka by Professor Dasgupta,[19] before the world came into being there was a "state devoid of all characteristics that is absolutely incoherent, indeterminate, and indefinite." This is the state of mutual equilibrium of guṇas called "avyakta." At some time – unpredictable and uncontrollable - a perturbation in avyakta took place with the resultant and unequal aggregation of latent guṇas and the start of a process of differentiation and heterogeneity. This process resulted sequentially in the development of mahat (buddhi/awareness), ahaṅkāra (individuation), and five bhūtas. These eight constituents beginning from avyakta and ending in pañcabhūtas are known as derivatives of prakṛti. In continuation, ten sense organs and mind appear followed by sense objects – a total of 16 derived from Prakṛti's evolutes (Figure 1). In infinite time, all that exists would dissolve into avyakta and the cosmic cycle would start again. There is no place for an external agent, a control, or a puruṣa in this entire cycle. This is the reason why the original sāṅkhya attributed to Caraka is regarded as "atheistic sāṅkhya." But yoga philosophy questioned how a "blind, non-intelligent" prakṛti could bring forth the order and harmony of the universe? How could it determine what course of evolution will be the best service to the puruṣas? How could it remove its own barriers and lend itself to the evolutionary process from the state of prakṛti equilibrium (avyakta)? The yoga line of argument concluded, "there must be some intelligent being who should help the course of evolution in such a way that this system or order and harmony may be attained. This Being is Īśvara."[20] This brought about the distinction between the seśvara-sāṅkhya (theistic sāṅkhya), and nirīśvara-sāṅkhya (atheistic sāṅkhya). Caraka's system with 24 constituents represented nirīśvara sāṅkhya, but the sound of Puruṣa is clearly heard in his description of self (ātma),[21] supreme self[22] and his enquiry into "The Body and its Knower."[23]

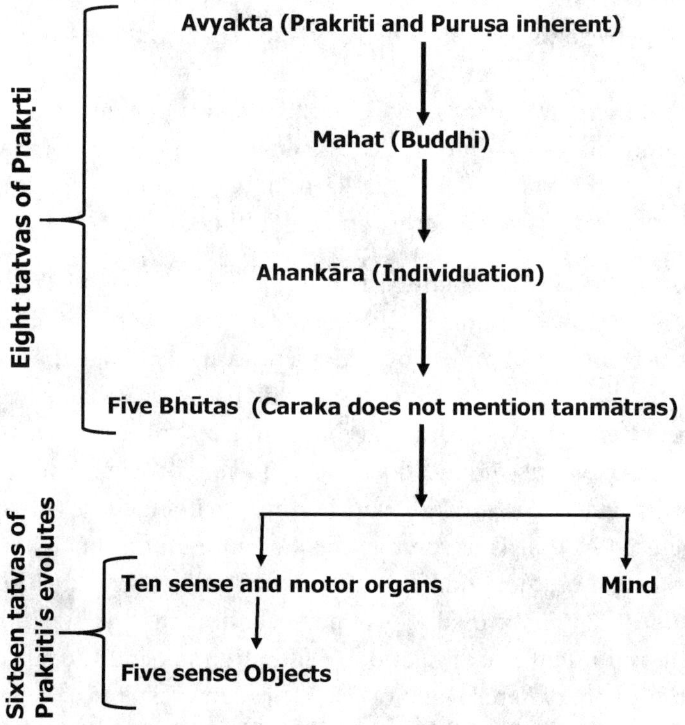

Figure 1: Evolution (pariṇāma) according to Caraka

Bhagavadgita had declared in no uncertain terms "this avyakta under discussion (sāṅkhya) is distinct from another avyakta which is eternal and independent of the appearance and disappearance of all animate and inanimate things."[24]

Human destiny

Is life span predetermined? This old question worried and tormented humans for ages but the patient and his physician felt its import more vividly. After all the patients' anxious query to the physician is not "what is my disease?" but "what would happen to me?" Caraka considered the subject of predestination and asked, "If life span is predetermined, where is the need or justification for mantras, oblations, auspicious rituals, propitiatory functions, and worship? Why should one steer clear of fierce beasts or fearful winds?"[25]

Reflections on life span led Caraka to adopt an enlightened and confident view towards the practice of medicine. Many people believe that serious illness and misery are caused by the effect of past Karma and no human effort can nullify the law of Karma; there are others who hold the view that we are ourselves responsible for our good or bad deeds and God rewards and decrees punishments accordingly; still others urge the Pauruṣeya view of Yoga Vāsiṣṭha that human will is all-powerful and there is no karmic or any other law which cannot be overcome by our own heroic effort. Among this welter, Caraka put forward an illuminating point of view[26] that stands out by its sweet reasonableness. According to him, life span is a product of the interplay of two forces – the effect of one's past deeds (daiva) and that of present actions. The forces may vary in strength, which would make the interplay mild, medium, or intense. A strong force of past deeds may overwhelm the force of present actions; on the other hand, a weak influence of past deeds may be neutralised by the strength of present actions. Unaware of this interplay of forces, some would claim that life span is predetermined, which need not be true in all circumstances. When appropriate action through adherence to the prescribed code of conduct overcomes the adverse effect of past deeds, the life span would be long, happy, and stable; if not, life would be short, unhappy, and unstable. When corrective actions and the efforts of past deeds are evenly matched, life span would be "neither too long nor too short."

If life span is not predetermined, Caraka went on, what is meant by timely and untimely death? He set forth the metaphor of a carriage and axle on which the wheels rotate. In course of time, the axle would wear out bit by bit and the carriage would fall apart from natural decay. The human body, if cared for properly, would similarly complete its life span when timely death would make its claim. If the axle breaks down due to overloading, bad road conditions, reckless driving, and non-lubrication, the carriage would break down prematurely. Similarly, individuals would die an untimely death due to over exertion, inappropriate food habits, abnormal body postures, sexual excess, suppression of natural urges, poisoning, fatal injuries caused by fire and wild animals, and treatment by incompetent physicians.[27]

Bio-ethics

In the grand oath administered by the Āchārya to students during initiation into a physician's training,[28] Caraka laid down an elaborate code of conduct, which covered the personal, professional, academic, social, and spiritual life of the candidate. It spared no aspect of medical ethics and remains a model oath even today. However, Caraka went beyond the domain of medical ethics when he drew special attention to the devastation of habitat by human activity.[29] He observed rulers presiding over cities and countries turning corrupt and dishonest, putting unjust pressure on officers, traders, and commoners until righteousness disappeared and "even gods took leave of the country." This was an invitation to all round shortages, starvation, and epidemics. He observed another kind of disaster when aggressive rulers unleashed wars out of greed and conceit, fleeced people with exorbitant taxes to conduct wars, caused many thousands of deaths and untold misery, and devastated the country.

According to Caraka, in both kinds of devastation, whatever may be the immediate cause, the ultimate cause is the violation of the rules of good conduct, which he had elaborated. He was vindicated by events in history. A tragic example was the plague in Manchuria, which killed a million people in the 19th century. The immediate cause of death of the victims was the plague bacillus – *Yersenia pestis* – but that does not represent the whole truth. In Manchuria, the wool from a rodent used to be harvested, which was highly prized by women in Europe for making shawls and coats. As Europe became rich in the 19th century, demand for the wool increased many-fold and the traders offered fancy prices for the wool in Manchuria. Tradition had forbidden the harvesting of wool from animals which were senile, sick looking, emaciated, or too young in Manchuria, but the lure of money overcame tradition and the local people began collecting wool from animals unmindful of restrictions. What was unknown at that time was the fact that the sick looking rodents were carriers of the causative bacillus!

When the aggressive harvesting of wool began, the organisms were released from the injured or dead rodents and they found unsuspecting hosts in thousands of labourers who developed bubonic plague which spread all over Manchuria and reached India. The immediate cause of the Manchurian plague was the organism of course but the colonial plunder by European nations, love of luxury of European women, greed of the traders, and the poor labourers who discarded age old customs for money were contributory causes and examples of unrighteous conduct as enunciated by Caraka. Just as many serious diseases in individuals are caused by errors of judgement and imprudent conduct (prajñāparādha), destruction of the habitat is brought about by the unrighteous conduct of the rulers and the ruled. Righteous conduct (sadvṛtti) should be the watchword for the individual and no less for the community.

An Āyurvedic view of Life

A study of Carakasaṃhitā gives one a ringside view of life. Indeed, CS had echoed *Mahābhārata*, "What you find here you may find elsewhere; but what you don't find here you will find nowhere." And the Āyurvedic view, while exalting lofty idealism, upholds the merits of a full life and signals the pathway to righteous living. The Āyurvedic view is a far cry from the Indian stereotype of indolence, pessimism, and extreme forms of renunciation.

Three urges of life: Caraka recognised three urges of all human endeavour, which stand in sharp contrast to the traditional disparagement of wealth and idolisation of renunciation. Caraka says,[30] "A person with a normal share of strength and combativeness, who is of sound mind and concern for things here and hereafter, is moved by three desires. These are the desire for life, for wealth, and for life hereafter. The desire for life comes first, because the loss of life amounts to the loss of everything. To ensure good life and health, the observance of a code of conduct is necessary, just as careful attention needs to be paid for the proper care of illness. The pursuit of wealth comes next, because wealth takes second place only to life. There is scarcely anything more miserable than a long life without the means to live. One should therefore work hard to make a living by engaging in farming, animal care, trade, service, and similar occupations. The third desire concerns life in another world after death, which does indeed raise many doubts."

The desire for long life in good health resonated throughout Caraka's code for living.[31] As described in Chapter 8, the code attached great importance to personal hygiene, nutrition, and tasty food, comfortable attire, jewellery, healthy social relations, and the pursuit of professional goals. While truthfulness, rectitude, courage, fearlessness, modesty, forgiveness, and kinship to all living beings were held supreme as virtues to be practiced, there was no bar on the celebration of life and the use of rasāyana and vājīkaraṇa to live for a hundred years and enjoy sexual vigour like a powerful horse!

The long and painstaking description of food and drinks, enjoyment of wine and even a wine party (Vāgbhaṭa) and the cheerful and confident attitude in Āyurvedic texts would convince the reader that, barring a small minority who were inclined to asceticism, their appeal was addressed to the great majority of people who sought to live a full and enjoyable life.

The second urge to earn wealth is self-evident because, as eloquently stated by Caraka, employment and earning a living by the "sweat of one's brow" were explicitly encouraged. The third urge consisted of a blissful afterlife. On this, Caraka conceded, there could be doubts as no "perceptible" evidence for afterlife could be advanced. However, he adroitly used this context to argue that knowledge could not always be reduced to what was perceptible as perception suffers from several limitations. By a series of epistemological arguments, Caraka established the validity of the urge to seek a blissful afterlife on the strength of the testimony of "aptas."

To be a physician: The choice of a physician's career was hailed and a good physician was revered as the guardian of life.[32] The oath administered to a trainee physician by the preceptor before a learned assembly enjoined him to the lifelong pursuit of knowledge, acquisition of skills, compassion to patients and all living beings, and a spotless conduct worthy of honour in personal and social life. A good physician would seek to acquire knowledge from shepherds and forest dwellers on medicinal plants, from the preceptor, scriptures, fellow students, and on his own from the accumulated experience of caring for patients. For the wise physician, the world would be a teacher[33] and his practice of medicine would be guided by compassion to fellow beings and not by self-aggrandisement or acquisition of wealth.

To live a good life: A good life must necessarily be virtuous but it must also be marked by right understanding and prudent action. Error in understanding and imprudent action - prajñāparādha - is responsible for causing a large number of diseases which are psychosomatic in origin and cannot be countered except by a conjoint approach of medical measures and righteous conduct. Medical measures could include dietary regime, physical activity, herbal formulations, and pañcakarma while righteous conduct would mandate self-control, non-violence, and good will for all creatures. Caraka's prescription for good conduct – Sadvṛtti – was most elaborate.[34] It insisted that a wholesome and healthy life could be achieved only if it was ethically compliant, and at the same time, mindful of prudent conduct at home, at work, and in the community.

References:

1. *CS Sūtra* 4: 23 - 29
2. *CS Sūtra* 1: 41 – 47
3. *CS Sūtra* 1: 58 – 62
4. *CS Sūtra* 1: 64 – 66
5. *CS Śārīra* 5: 5
6. *CS Śārīra* 5: 10 – 11
7. S N Gupta. *A History of Indian Philosophy*, Motilal Banarasidas, Delhi 1997. Vol 1: Page 280.
8. *CS Sūtra* 1: 41

9. *CS Sūtra* 1: 48 – 52
10. S N Gupta. *A History of Indian Philosophy*, Motilal Banarasidas, Delhi 1997. Vol 1: Page 332-333.
11. *CS Sūtra* 11: 18 – 19
12. *CS Vimāna* 4: 6
13. *CS Vimāna* 4: 3 – 8
14. *CS Sūtra* 11: 23 – 24
15. *CS Vimāna* 8
16. *CS Vimāna* 8: 27 – 66
17. S N Gupta. *A History of Indian Philosophy*, Motilal Banarasidas, Delhi 1997. Vol II: Page 399
18. *CS Śārīra* 1: 18 – 23
19. S N Gupta. *A History of Indian Philosophy*, Motilal Banarasidas, Delhi 1997. Vol 1: Page 213
20. S N Gupta. *A History of Indian Philosophy*. Motilal Banarasidas, Delhi 1997. Vol 1: Page 258 – 259
21. *CS Śārīra* 1: 39 – 44
22. *CS Śārīra* 1: 53
23. M S Valiathan *The Legacy of Caraka*, Orient Blackswan, Chennai 2003. Page 184 – 188.
24. *BG* 8: 20
25. M S Valiathan *The Legacy of Caraka*, Orient Blackswan, Chennai 2003. Page 153.
26. *CS Vimāna* 3: 29 – 32
27. *CS Vimāna* 3: 38
28. *CS Vimāna* 8: 13 – 14
29. *CS Vimāna* 3: 6 -7
30. *CS Sūtra* 11: 3 - 8
31. *CS Sūtra* 5: 71 – 75
32. *CS Sūtra* 9: 18
33. *CS Vimāna* 8: 14
34. *CS Sūtra* 1: 8

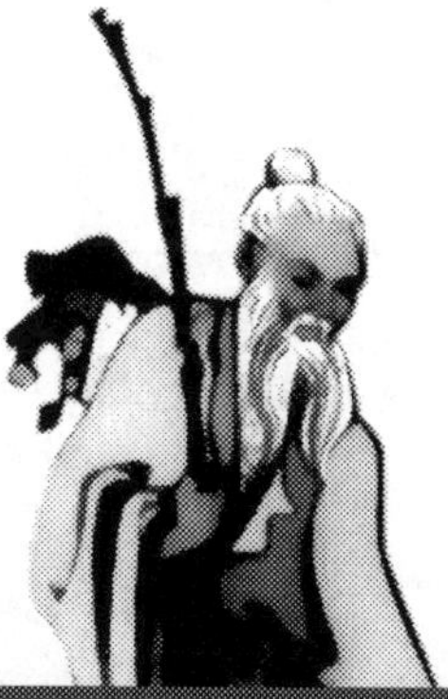

CHAPTER 5

Body in Health

In the training of physicians, the first year is largely spent in learning basic medical sciences, which consist of anatomy, physiology, and biochemistry. This has become universal as modern understanding of medicine everywhere is increasingly based on the foundation of basic sciences and its practice is evidence-based. In India, even the training of physicians in Āyurvedic colleges begins with the basic science subjects listed above. In ancient India, the training of physicians was however carried out in Gurukulas spread all over the country and in a few great universities. Anatomy was well known and recognised as an essential subject in a physician's training by Suśruta and Caraka. Suśruta also recommended dissection of cadavers as a practical method of learning anatomy. We have already seen in Viśuddhi Magga and other Buddhist literature that teachers and physicians in Buddhist India used anatomical knowledge in medical practice. But the knowledge of physiology and biochemistry then was imperfect not only in India but also in contemporary civilisations in Europe and China. The approach used in learning the three basic subjects in a physician's training in ancient India was to focus on the structure and functions of the whole body in a healthy state. This was inescapable as the knowledge - of organs, viscera, and tissues based on detailed dissection in anatomy; of the functions of various organs and systems in physiology; and of the chemical events associated with physiological activity in biochemistry was defective. In this chapter, an effort will be made to see how the students of Āyurveda in ancient India understood the human body in health by focusing attention on selected themes from the texts of Caraka and Suśruta.

It is interesting to recall that the structure of the human body received attention in the Atharvaveda, which inspired Āyurveda. The Sūkta "The Wonderful Structure of Man"[1] consists of questions on the joints, limbs, trunk, bones, jaws, brain, and other organs but also on life breath, success, truth, wisdom, and music, which go far beyond structure. The questions were always couched in earnest phraseology "Who designed it? Who made it? Who brought together the arms to do acts of heroism?" No wonder Āyurveda followed the trail blazed by the "Wonderful Structure of Man"!

Body in Health - Structure:

Structure signifies form and includes the body, its parts, organs, tissues, body fluids, bones and joints and the entire physical frame of an individual. The following themes relating to structure, which received serious attention in the ancient texts would enable the reader to visualise the "big picture" of the body in health which interested physicians in ancient India. The themes are:

- Foetal development;
- Body Parts;
- Organs; and
- Vital spots (Marmas).

Foetal development:

This was a theme, which received much attention even before Āyurveda laid emphasis on it. Not only did India's epics Rāmāyaṇa and Bhāgavata refer to it in some detail but even an earlier Upaniṣad - Garbhopaniṣad – associated with Atharvaveda gave a detailed explanation on the evolution of the embryo in the mother's womb. Paul Deussen regarded the Upaniṣad to be "more like a manual on physiology or medicine than a spiritual text!"

In Āyurveda, the union of the male and female seeds following sexual intercourse signals the formation of the embryo. The foetus consists of contributions from the parents, nutrients in the uterine environment, and self, which enters the foetus through the medium of the mind in the third month. Defects in the male or female seeds, effect of past actions – Karma, uterine environment, and mother's nutrition – all these could affect the growth and development of foetus and result in foetal anomalies.

A distinctive view of Āyurveda in embryogenesis and foetal development was the identification of the derivatives of the original constituents of embryo in the developing foetus. According to this hypothesis, the contributions of the mother, father, self, nutrition, mind, and congeniality to the developing foetus can be identified (Table 1).

Table 1: Individual contributions to foetal development

Contributor	Contribution to Foetal Development
Mother	Soft tissues; viscera
Father	Hard tissues including bone, teeth, ligaments, hair
Self	Entry into the united seed vitalizes the foetus; causes birth in higher species, endows self-knowledge, life span, consciousness, and will
Nutrition	Growth and consolidation of the body, energy, maintenance of breathing
Mind	Enters in conjunction with self; supports sense organs; source of tendencies, conduct, likes, memory, courage, and fear
Congeniality	Congeniality in food and lifestyle between father and mother determines good health, cheerfulness, fine voice, and fertility of individual.

The belief that soft tissues and hard tissues in the foetus were derived from the maternal and paternal seeds would imply that diseases affecting those tissues would have a genetic origin. The influence of mother's nutrition and her cheerful and positive attitude on foetal growth was also recognised. High value was attached to the compatibility in food and lifestyle between the mother and father for the healthy development of the foetus.

Ancient physicians had made observations on the time "horizons" of foetal development (Table 2).

Table 2: Time "horizons" of foetal development

Month	Foetal Development
First	A shapeless mass; all constituents endowed with all the qualities of five elements
Second	Solidifies as a bolus; solid, flesh-like, and tumour-like appearances suggest male, female, and neuter gender
Third	Head/heart/navel/sense organs/rectum as the start controversial. Another view was that the first organ to develop could not be settled because it is not observable. The consensus was all organs develop simultaneously. The organs traceable to their origin from five elements. Body parts including sense organs appear; consciousness makes entry; maternal and foetal hearts connected and emotions resonate, hence maternal cravings ("pica")

Month	Foetal Development
Fourth	Umbilical cord attached to the navel at one end and placenta at the other; opposite side of placenta connected to mother's heart, which soaks the placenta with blood through pulsating vessels; foetal head up in the uterus; face to the back of the mother and limbs folded. The head rotates and comes down only at delivery.
Fifth	Development of flesh and blood progresses rapidly
Sixth	Mother's strength and complexion decrease: those of foetus improve
Seventh	Mother wears out: foetus strong
Eighth	Ebb and flow of ojas between mother and foetus and transport of rasas nourish the foetus but weaken mother. Delivery during this month is risky.
Ninth	Ninth to tenth is the time for parturition – longer intrauterine stay of foetus harmful.

It is clear that ancient physicians could not have made these observations without closely examining the aborted foetuses and correlating them with the duration of pregnancy. What is of great interest is the observation that consciousness enters the foetus in the third month, which has an important bearing on the termination of pregnancy today and its legal and ethical implications. It is interesting that the hearts of mother and foetus beating in unison (dauhṛdam) in the third month could have suggested a connection with "pica" – the desire to eat sour or sweet items which the mother may not have desired before – as it could be a reflection of the vicarious desire of the foetus! In Āyurveda, heart is the seat of emotions and intellect. The vigorous debate on foetal development as vividly recorded in CS shows the great importance attached to this subject in Āyurveda.

Foetal anomalies were traced to maternal and paternal factors, which were genetic; they were also traced to maternal nutrition and life style, which were environmental factors. The effect of Karma was also recognised as a cause because many congenital anomalies defied explanations based on genetics or environment. Āyurveda recognised personality types – sātvika, rājasika, and tāmasika – as determined at conception. This does influence the individual's predisposition to diseases as well as the response to treatment.

Body parts:

The clearest description of body parts – anatomy – is given by Suśruta in an entire chapter.[2] While this chapter enumerates body parts, organs, joints, bones, and so on, detailed descriptions of individual organs are more likely to be found elsewhere in the Saṃhitā, where that specific organ is being discussed in relation to a disease or a surgical procedure. For example, rectum would be found listed in this chapter but its detailed structure will be found in the chapter on Piles. It was felt that a physician in training should possess sound knowledge of body parts but details of specific organs like eye, urinary bladder, or rectum need be the concern of specialists even in those far-off days!

Suśruta's description of body parts, sub-parts, body constituents, bones, ligaments, and muscles is given in Tables 3 to 8.[3] Bones are discussed in greater detail because of special interest.

Table 3: Body parts and sub-parts

Parts	Sub-parts	
Head and neck (1)	Head and Neck	Head top (cranium); forehead; nose; chin; neck (one each) ears, eyes, eyebrows, temples, cheeks (two each).
Upper limbs (2)	Upper limbs	Shoulders, axillae, upper arms, elbows (two each), fingers (ten).
Lower limbs (2)	Lower limbs	Groin, hips, thighs, knees (two each), toes (ten)
Trunk (1)	Trunk	Abdomen, back, umbilicus, urinary bladder (one each), breasts, sides, testicles, (two each)

Table 4: Body constituents

Body constituents	Numbers	Description
Twak	7	Layers
Kalā	7	Membranes
Āśaya	7	Viscera
Dhātus	7	Tissues
Śiras	700	Blood vessels
Pēśi	500	Muscles
Snāyu	900	Ligaments
Asthi	300	Bones
Sandhi	210	Joints
Marmas	107	Vital spots
Dhamani	24	Large vessels
Doṣa	3	Vāta, pitta, kapha
Mala	3	Execrable
Dvāras	9	Natural openings
Kaṇḍara	16	Tendons
Jāla	16	Networks
Kūrcas	6	Brush like hair
Rajju	4	Fasciae/sheath

Body constituents	Numbers	Description
Sevanī	7	Raphe
Saṅghāta	14	Joints where several bones are articulated
Sīmanta	14	In the above, the suture lines constitute sīmanta
Yogavāhasrotas	24	Body channels
Āntra	2	Intestines

Table 5: Joints

Location	Number
a. Extremities	68
b. Trunk	59
c. Above the neck	83
Total	**210**

Table 6: Ligaments (Snāyu)

Parts	Number
Toes	30 (6 per toe)
Sole, Tarsus, Ankle	30
Leg	30
Knee	10
Thigh	40
Hip	10
Sub Total for two legs	**150**
Total for 4 extremities*	**600**
*The same pattern and numbers are applicable to lower and upper extremities.	
Lumbar region	60
Back	80
Sides	60
Chest	30
Neck	36
Head	34
Grand Total	**900**

Table 7: Muscle

Location	Number
a. Extremities	400
b. Trunk	66
c. Neck and above	34
Total	**500**

Bones: Caraka mentioned the total number of bones in the body as 360, which was in conformity with the number given in the Atharvaveda. Suśruta explicitly differed from the Vedic total and gave his total as 300.

Table 8: Bones (Asthi)

Part/Sub-part	Number of bones	Total
Leg		
Toe	3	15
Sole, tarsus, ankle	10	10
Heel	1	1
Leg	2	2
Knee	1	1
Thigh	1	1
a. Two Legs: Sub Total		**60**
b. Two Arms (Same enumeration as legs): Sub Total		**60**
Pelvis		
Anus, perineum, hips	4	4
Sacrum	1	1
c. Pelvis: Sub Total		**5**
Side	36	72
d. Side: Sub Total		**72**
Back	30	30
e. Back: Sub Total		**30**
Chest	8	8
f. Chest: Sub Total		**8**
Scapular region	2	2
g. Scapular region: Sub Total		**2**
h. Neck and above:		
Neck	9	9
Air passage	4	4
Jaw	2	2
Teeth	32	32
Nose	3	3
Palate	1	1
Cheek	1	2
Ear	1	2
Temple	1	2
Skull	6	6
Neck and above Sub Total		**63**
Total: [a+b+c+d+e+f+g+h]		**300**

The total number of bones in modern anatomy is 200, the big increase in the older total being largely due to the practice of counting cartilages, teeth, and bony protuberances as bones.

Unlike bones, cartilages and hard tissues, muscles, fascia, viscera, etc., were inaccurately described and enumerated. The total number of muscles, according to Suśruta, was 487 whereas the correct number today is 213. The reason for this discrepancy lies in the practice of dissection in Suśruta's period, when it was done in cadavers in the early stage of rotting in shallow waters by scraping off one layer after the next with sharp edges of leaves or splinters.[4] There were obviously strong taboos against touching, leave aside cutting, of cadavers in ancient India.

Organs:

Body constituents (Table 4) refer to seven āśayas, which are viscera. These include lung (kaphāśaya, puphusa), gall bladder (pittāśaya), heart (raktāśaya), stomach (āmāśaya), intestines (āntra), urinary bladder (mūtrāśaya), and uterus in women (garbhāśaya). Caraka lists fifteen in a grouping called "koṣṭāṅga," which includes viscera as shown below:[5]

Umbilicus (Nābhī)	Heart (Hṛdayam)
Lung (Kloma)	Liver (Yakṛt)
Spleen (Plīha)	Kidney (vṛkka)
Urinary bladder (Vasti)	Caecum (Purīṣādhāra)
Stomach (Āmāśaya)	Jejunum (Pakvāśaya)
Rectum (Uttaraguda)	Anus (Adharaguda)
Small intestine (Kṣudranthra)	Large intestine (Sthūlanthra)
Omentum (Vapāvahara)	

One can note several differences between the classifications and nomenclature of Suśruta and Caraka in regard to viscera. Suśruta restricted the term to āśayas or organs, which served as receptacles whereas Caraka included them among internal organs (koṣṭāṅga). Though the locations of these organs were known and their main functions were vaguely known, there were two major omissions. The function of the lung (puphusa, kloma, terminology varies) was not known even though the inspiration–expiration sequence and the role of life breath (prāṇa) were well recognised. Secondly, brain is not mentioned in this list though "mastiṣka" in the skull is mentioned elsewhere. More importantly its function is not mentioned anywhere. The location and external appearance of the heart, its connection to ten vessels and content of blood were known, but its interior of four chambers was unknown. Obviously, the knowledge of the anatomy of internal organs and soft parts of the body in general remained highly defective due to the unsatisfactory method of cadaveric dissection in Suśruta's time and its total disappearance subsequently.

Vital spots *(Marmas):*

Vital spots or marma is a unique concept in Āyurvedic anatomy even though the term finds mention in the Ṛigveda. As the term implies, injury to the spots was attended by death or serious disability; secondly, injury included surgical incisions or puncture for blood-letting, which had to spare them at all costs. A vital spot is a point of assemblage of muscle, blood vessel, ligaments, bone and joint, where life breath was believed to reside.[6] The spot could be dominated by one of the five structures in the list as indicated below:[7]

Dominating structures	**Number of Marmas**
Muscle	11
Blood vessels	41
Ligaments	27
Bone	8
Joints	20
Total	**107**

The distribution of the vital spots and their exact location in the upper and lower extremities, chest, abdomen, back, head, and neck were described in detail. Apart from this classification, they were also grouped based on prognosis following injuries as follows:[8]

- Instantly fatal;
- Fatal after days;
- Fatal following the removal of a foreign body;
- Cause of deformity and disability; and
- Cause of insufferable pain.

The gravity of injury to many spots is immediately obvious such as a spot on the precordium "between the two breasts and above the pit of the stomach"; death or disability after several days could be due to infection or injury to nerves. Death following the removal of a foreign body could be due to severe bleeding from an artery, which had been plugged or, after an interval of several days, due to gas gangrene. However, a good many among the 107 vital spots are hard to explain in terms of the grave prognosis following injury.

Along with other manipulative and surgical procedures for treating fractures and dislocations and various surgical conditions, practice based on vital spots also virtually disappeared from the mainstream of Āyurveda by the fourth or fifth centuries of CE. In the practice of medicine by Vaidyas, vital spots or marmas had little role or importance. However, just as the setting of fractures and surgical procedures disappeared from the mainstream of Āyurveda, only to reappear and survive among traditional practitioners who had no formal training in Āyurveda, practice based on vital spots became the focal point and basis of a system of physical therapy, especially in Kerala, where its influence on the evolution of martial arts was also considerable.

Body in Health: Functions

The discussion above focused on the structure of the body in health. The present section will provide a complementary view of functions which sustain the body in good health. It is based on the teachings and cues from the texts of Caraka and Suśruta as follows:

- Sāmya;
- Digestion;
- Tridoṣa doctrine;
- Circulation of Blood; and
- Nervous system.

Sāmya

In terms of body function, a generalisation of great importance is the concept of sāmya, which can be translated as equilibrium. It impinges on every aspect of body function in so far as the equilibrium of various components and functions in the body is essential for the maintenance of good health. The equilibrium is however not unitary and is a conglomeration of equilibrium of several components and functions of the body. Āyurveda regards sāmya as a synonym of health and its opposite, vaiṣamya as that of ill health. Consider these sāmyas:

Dhātusāmya:[9] Seven dhātus – rasa, blood, muscle, adipose tissue, bone, marrow, and semen -are the constituents of the body and they are required to maintain equilibrium among themselves and with the rest of the body.

Doṣasāmya:[10] Doṣas vāta, pitta, and kapha are malas or execrables which are by-products of the digestive processes taking place in the dhātus all the time. Within limits these three malas are necessary and are regarded as dhātus (maladhātus), which must be in equilibrium among themselves and with the rest of the body. When the limits are breached, the equilibrium is disturbed. The resulting disequilibrium is disease.

Agnisāmya:[11] Digestion is a constant and never ending activity in body constituents and body parts including the stomach and gut. Digestion is performed by agnis (fire) wherever it takes place, the most prominent of agnis being the one which functions in the stomach. All these fires must be in equilibrium as any breach leading to disequilibrium would cause body dysfunction and disease.

Ṛtusāmya:[12] Body must be in equilibrium with the changing seasons and has in-built mechanisms such as sweating and shivering to restore thermal equilibrium in response to environmental changes. When these mechanisms cease to work or the seasonal changes are extreme, disequilibrium occurs leading to disease conditions such as heat stroke.

Hetusāmya: Hetu means cause and with reference to disease it means the cause of a disease. The causes abound within and around the body all the time and there is no way they can be eliminated and the body and surroundings sanitised. Nonetheless people remain well because the causes within their body and in the surroundings, have developed a state of equilibrium with the body of the subjects. The presence of causes within the body does not necessarily mean disease which occurs only when the equilibrium breaks down and the quiescent cause becomes active.[13] The aim of therapy is to bring back equilibrium, by promoting dhātus which are in equilibrium and by giving up things which promote disequilibrium.[14]

The collective equilibrium or sāmya as the physiological basis of health is analogous to Claude Bernard's famous postulation of "constant internal environment" as a necessary condition of healthy living.

Digestion

Among the vital functions of the body such as respiration, blood circulation, digestion of food, urinary secretion and neurological regulation of body functions, digestion of food was dealt with in the greatest detail in Āyurveda. Digestion (dīpana) was believed to take place mainly in the stomach but also in all the seven dhātus of the body round the clock.[15] The agent to energise the digestive process is agni, which is specific to the location such as stomach, muscle, or bone. Among the agnis, the one in the stomach (jaṭharāgni) is pre-eminent. The waxing and waning of the agnis have a profound effect on not only health but also life itself.

Food and drinks which reach the stomach are acted upon by jaṭharāgni and subjected to churning by wind (samāna).[16] As a result, two products emerge which are āhāra rasa and kitta. Āhāra rasa is the large fraction, which goes to different body constituents to replenish them while kitta is the remainder, which gets eliminated. The movement of āhāra rasa and kitta through body channels is powered by two different winds – vyāna and apāna, which are parts of prāṇa or life breath. From the stomach, āhāra rasa passes into the duodenum (pakvāśaya) where it is joined by bile (pitta). As āhāra rasa and kitta travel in the gut, their paths diverge. Āhāra rasa turns into a finer product (sūkṣmabhāga) "rasa" which would nourish depleting dhātus, whereas kitta would be desiccated and associated with apāna for expulsion through the anus.

The course of finer product - rasa (Figure 1) represents the core of the Āyurvedic concept of digestion. From the gut, rasa passes through channels called dhamanis to the heart; from there it reaches the liver which imparts bile to it, when the red coloured blood makes its appearance.

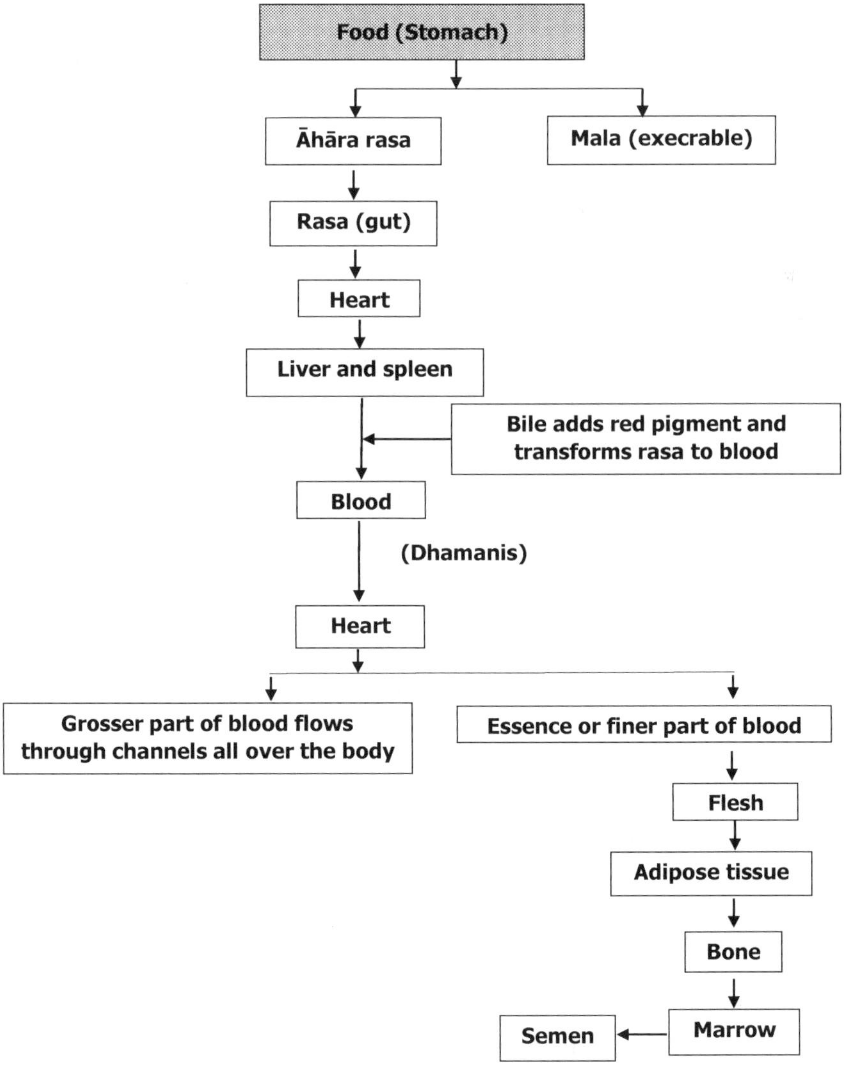

Figure 1: Course of Āhāra Rasa

A "waste product" which appears during the rasa to blood transformation is kapha of tridoṣa; blood goes back to the heart through dhamanis. The large portion of blood (sthūlabhaga) flows out of the heart to get distributed all over the body through countless channels; a finer portion (sūkṣmabhāga) follows a different course. This part transforms into flesh when a waste product also appears, which is pitta - one of the three doṣas. Sequentially, the finer portion of muscle transforms into adipose tissue, when the waste products such as earwax are also produced. Adipose tissue transforms into bone, when sweat appears as waste product, and bone turns to marrow, when the "waste product" is vāta. The essence of marrow transforms into semen. Tridoṣa – vāta, pitta, and kapha - are products of digestion which are not assimilable but which are of critical importance. Within their normal range, the three doṣas are regarded as dhātus (mala dhātus) and are essential for the normal functioning of the body (doṣasāmya); when their normal proportions are breached by excess or deficiency (doṣavaisāmya), illness results. The sequential transformations in dhātus are effected by agnis specific to each dhātu. The cascade of transformations from rasa to semen is believed to complete in one month.[17]

Tridoṣa doctrine

Vāta, pitta, and kapha as digestive products: The doctrine of vāta, pitta, and kapha dominates the theory and practice of Āyurveda. As their genesis is inseparable from the digestive process, it is appropriate at this stage to discuss the tridoṣa doctrine.

Kitta – the execrable part of the products of digestion in the gut – and execrables such as ear wax resulting from the digestive process in the dhātus which are eliminated, other execrables called malas which result from the digestive action in the dhātus have a physiological role in Āyurveda. They are designated as "mala-dhātus" as long as their proportions to the dhātus are maintained. Vāta, pita, and kapha are the most important among mala-dhātus and the maintenance of their equilibrium is indispensable for health. If their levels fall below the range, they need to be restored by fresh inputs; and if their level becomes excess, therapeutic measures are called for to evacuate the excess. The śodhana measures are often employed by physicians to correct the excess accumulation of doṣas. The origin of the three doṣas from the metabolism of food, the sequential replenishment of dhātus, the role of malas and the special status of vāta, pitta, and kapha are shown in (Figure 2).

Doṣa-dominated constitution of individuals (doṣa prakṛti): If the disequilibrium of doṣas is the beginning of disease, could a doṣa-dominated constitution be prone to the incidence of diseases? This was a legitimate question especially because Āyurveda recognised that three primary constitutional types – vāta, pitta, and kapha – are fixed at the time of the conception of the embryo.[18] This was important because, according to Āyurveda, the constitutional type determines an individual's predisposition to disease as well as his/her response to treatment. The determination of the constitutional type of individuals is made by physicians on the basis of their physical, mental, and behavioural traits.[19] Recent investigations, have shown that doṣaprakṛti has indeed a genomic basis.[20]

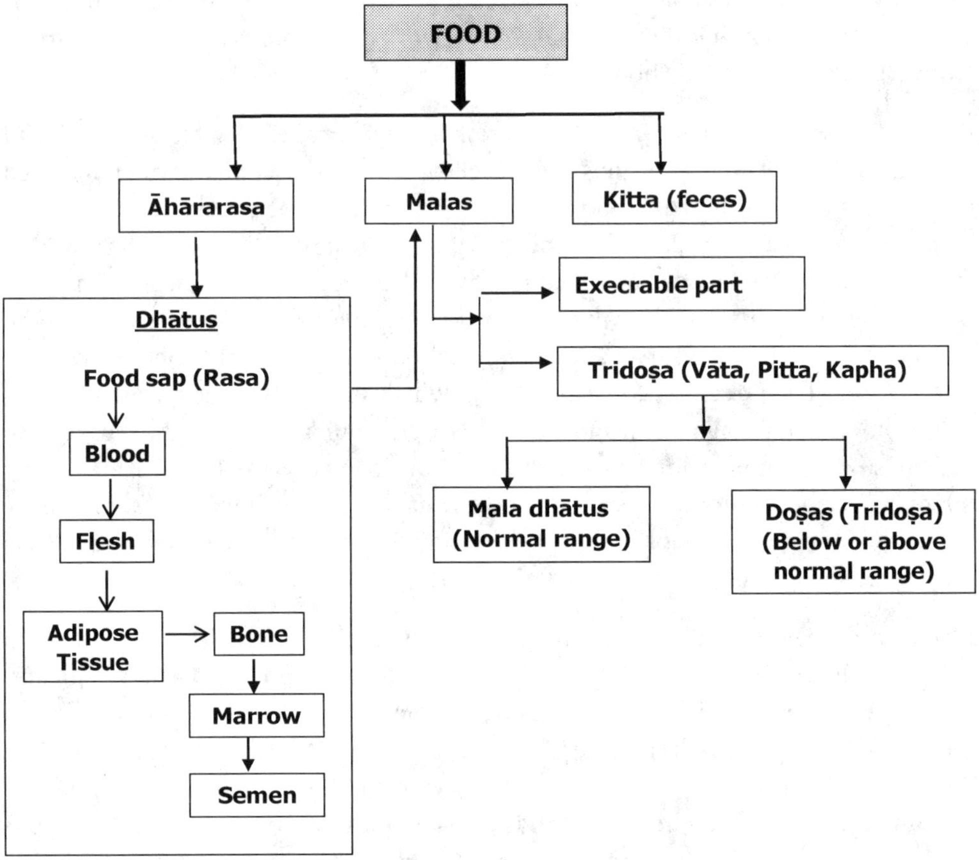

Figure 2: Origin of Tridoṣa

Circulation of blood:

Blood vessels: Heart, blood vessels, and blood flow were recognised and described by Caraka and Suśruta. Suśruta's descriptions are clearer and more detailed in regard to heart and blood vessels. According to him, heart has the shape of a lotus bud, hanging with the apex facing downward.[21] He held that rasa – the finer part of āhāra rasa – runs through the whole body and has its primary location in the heart, whence it flows through 24 vessels which originate from the heart and ramify toward every part of the body.[22] There is much confusion regarding "vessels" which include sirās, dhamani, nāḍī, and srota. Suśruta claims that of the 24 dhamanis, ten course upwards, ten downwards and four around the body. Their subdivisions are given as those carrying vāta, pitta, kapha, blood, rasa, śabda, rūpa, gandha, sound, and induction to sleep and for waking up, tears, breast milk and semen. Subdivisions of the ten dhamanis coursing upwards functionally bind the upper and lower halves of the body.[23] Similar classifications are given for the dhamanis coursing downwards and around the body. It is obvious that this network of dhamanis cannot be regarded as a vascular system of the body.

Heart: We find no description of the interior of the heart in the texts of Caraka and Suśruta. As far as its function goes, it was believed to be a receptacle, which received three kinds of fluid – rasa, blood, and ojas, heart being the primary seat of rasa; blood, as noted earlier, reached the heart from the liver; ojas is a yellowish fluid of critical importance, the loss of which is fatal.[24] These three vital fluids reach every part of the body through the vessels carrying various names. Heart supports the structure and functions of the entire body as a house is supported by pillars and rafters.[25] Heart is the seat of consciousness,[26] which sustains the proper functioning of the mind, soul, cognition, and emotions. The soul resides in the heart. The channels or dhamanis connected to the heart are two-way conduits because, they not only transport fluids away from the heart but also convey impulses from all over the body to the heart. The blockage of the conduits through which mind operates is the immediate cause of insanity.[27]

Blood circulation: The movement of blood and body fluids through body channels is a recurring theme in ancient Indian literature. The Kena sūkta - "The Wonderful Structure of Man" - of the Atharvaveda had in fact referred to "flow in rivers pink, rosy red, and coppery dark running in all ways in man and upwards and downwards". From the descriptions in Caraka and more clearly in Suśruta, one can claim that rasa and blood enter the heart, which is already the seat of ojas. These three vital fluids would seem to enjoy some form of flow separation in the heart, which has apparently only one chamber. Furthermore, blood is derived from rasa, and ojas, according to Caraka, is derived from semen as the ultimate product of the evolution of dhātus. Heart serves as a receptacle of the three fluids, which exit from it through a variety of channels to all the dhātus in the body far and near.

Nowhere is there a mention of heart as a pump or these fluids returning from their destinations to the heart in any form. The heart receives refills of rasa and blood as the products of the non-stop digestive process in the stomach and dhātus. Though heart serves as a receptacle from which rasa and blood flow towards all parts of the body and receives refills of rasa and blood from the normal process of digestion, this can hardly be called the circulation of blood. From Suśruta's metaphor of a tank for holding water for irrigation and the channels on the ground keeping the field moist and fruitful, it would seem that heart was seen as a reservoir and its various conduits as channels to supply the dhātus. The tank is not refilled by the water consumed by returning from the crops in the field, but by fresh supplies from external sources.

Respiration:

In contrast to the digestion of food and circulation of blood, references to respiration are scanty and too brief in Caraka and Suśruta. This did not constrain them from giving detailed descriptions of the clinical features and treatment of lung diseases such as tuberculosis and bronchial asthma. The lung (kloma/puphusa) was known but its function seems to have been unknown; trachea (mahāsrota/kanṭhanāḍī) was mentioned by Caraka in discussing laboured breathing.[28] There are also references to the compartmentalisation of life breath (prāṇa) and udāna (chest and throat), vāyu in inhalation and exhalation and speech.[29] These somewhat disjointed references indicate the limited understanding of the life-sustaining role of respiration and the functions of the lung.

The rudimentary knowledge about respiration in the medical texts contrasts with the yoga literature, including Patañjali's yoga sūtra, which deals with Aṣṭāṅga yoga and its practice as a means of self-realization. One of the crucial steps recommended by the sūtra for the student of yoga is breath control which involves not only a sound understanding of the technique but also the mechanism of action of breath control and its effect on the body and the mind. Āyurveda took no notice of yogic literature on breath control which undoubtedly existed in the first century CE when Caraka is believed to have lived.

Nervous system: [30, 31]

Though "brain" was located in the skull and mentioned thrice in CS, its function was not indicated in CS or SS. The general term "śirā" (head) was often used as a vital part (uthamāṅga), in which life breath inheres and to which all senses belong, but there was no mention of the brain having any role in it. Suśruta[32] refers to four dhamanis in the neck on either side of the trachea (kanṭhanāḍī) and injury to any of them producing dumbness, hoarseness and loss of taste. He also refers to two nerves on the back of the ear, injury to which would produce deafness: two on either side of the nasal aperture, injury to which would produce loss of smell, and two nerves on the back of the eyebrows, damage to which would cause blindness. He clearly mentions that the cognitive nerves are attached to the brain, but, like Caraka, he considered the heart as the only seat of consciousness. The impossibility of distinguishing sira, dhamanis, and nāḍī in the ancient descriptions seriously impedes a study of the nervous system. Suśruta refers to the cranial nerves mentioned above as "sira," but venesection is (siravedha) also done in sira! The only ancient authority who recognised brain as the seat of consciousness was Bhela who was a fellow student of Agniveśa under Ācrāya Ātreya, whose treatise was redacted by Caraka several centuries later.

An abiding mystery is why Āyurveda took no notice of the ideas in relation to consciousness in the yoga system which was no less ancient. Patañjali is believed to have composed the yoga sūtras in the second century BCE (Dasgupta), which explicitly links consciousness with the brain and the central nervous system. Caraka was aware of Patañjali's yoga as he refers to various siddhis of yoga.[33] Though every new doctrine was challenged and debates were strongly encouraged, barriers seem to have existed inexplicably between knowledge systems as illustrated by the walls which existed between Āyurveda and Yoga in the understanding of respiration and of cognitive functions in ancient India.

References:

1. *AV*, X. 2
2. *SS Śārīra*, 5
3. *CS Śārīra*, 5: 4 – 38 – 45
4. *SS Śārīra*, 5: 42 – 51
5. *CS Śārīra*, 7: 10
6. *SS Śārīra*, 6: 3
7. *SS Śārīra*, 6: 4
8. *SS Śārīra*, 6: 17
9. *CS Sūtra*, 1: 53
10. *CS Sūtra*, 13: 13
11. *CS Vimāna*, 6: 12
12. *CS Sūtra*, 6: 3
13. *CS Nīdana*, 4: 4
14. *CS Sūtra*, 16: 34 - 38
15. *CS Sūtra*, 28: 3
16. *CS Sūtra*, 28: 4 - 5
17. *SS Sūtra*, 14: 15
18. *CS Vimāna*, 8: 95
19. *CS Vimāna*, 96 - 98

20. Genome-wide analysis correlates *Āyurveda prakṛti*, Periyasamy Govindaraj, Sheikh Nizamuddin, Anugula Sharath, Vuskamalla Jyothi, Harish Rotti, Ritu Raval, Jayakrishna Nayak, Balakrishna K Bhat, BV Prasanna, Pooja Shintre, Mayura Sule, Kalpana S Joshi, Amrish P Dedge, Ramachandra Bharadwaj, GG Gangadharan, Sreekumaran Nair, Puthiya M Gopinath, Bhushan Patwardhan, Paturu Kondaiah, Kapaettu Satyamoorthy, Marthanda Varma Sankaran Valiathan and Kumarasamy Thangaraj. Nature Communications, Scientific Reports, 5:15786, DOI: 10.1038/srep15786 (2015).
21. *SS*, III. 4 – 32
22. *SS Sūtra*, 14: 3
23. *SS*, III. 4 – 30
24. *CS Sūtra*, 17: 74
25. *CS Sūtra*, 30: 4
26. *CS Śārīra*, 7: 10
27. *CS Nidāna*, 7: 4
28. *CS Vimāna*, 5: 5
29. *CS Sūtra*, 18: 55
30. *CS Siddhi*, 9: 79
31. *Cikitsā*, 26: 105
32. *SS Śārīra*, 6: 66 – 75
33. *CS Śārīra*, 1: 140 - 141

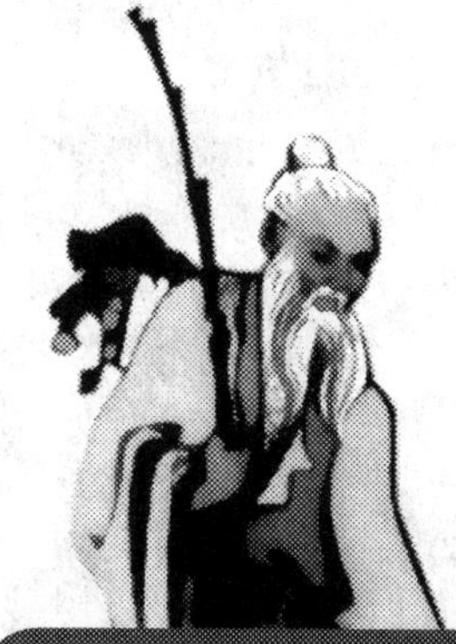

CHAPTER 6

Body in Disease

For all his devotion to philosophy, Caraka redacted Agniveśa's Tantra to provide an authoritative text on diseases and their treatment. From a recent exercise in archeo-epidemiology based on the descriptions in CS,[1] we see darkly through a cloud of many centuries that infectious diseases were much more common in Caraka's India than non-infectious conditions, and physicians were well aware of the capabilities and limitations of medical practice. Caraka, for example, enjoins the physician to determine whether the disease of the patient is curable, curable with difficulty, or incurable before starting therapy.[2] Obviously, there were many diseases beyond cure in his days as there are now 2000 years later. He, however, urged physicians to keep in mind that an individual's existence is based on the body, which must be protected under all circumstances.[3, 4]

Though Āyurvedic texts deal with diseases and their management extensively, Āyurveda regarded health as the natural state of humans and disease as an aberration. Even if an aberration or deviation from the natural state should occur, the natural tendency would reassert and restore normalcy sooner or later. This was a common observation. As the Chinese pilgrim Hieun Tsiang noted, patients in India seemed to recover from common illness by fasting for seven days and, if that did not work, they would consult a physician. Vāgbhaṭa likened a physician's role to give a helping hand to a sufferer who is mired in the muck of disease[5] (Figure 1). The inherent tendency to remain well and get out of illness on one's own had been observed by the Atharvaveda which called upon the "healing creepers" eaten by pigs, mongoose, and snakes during illness to protect them.[6]

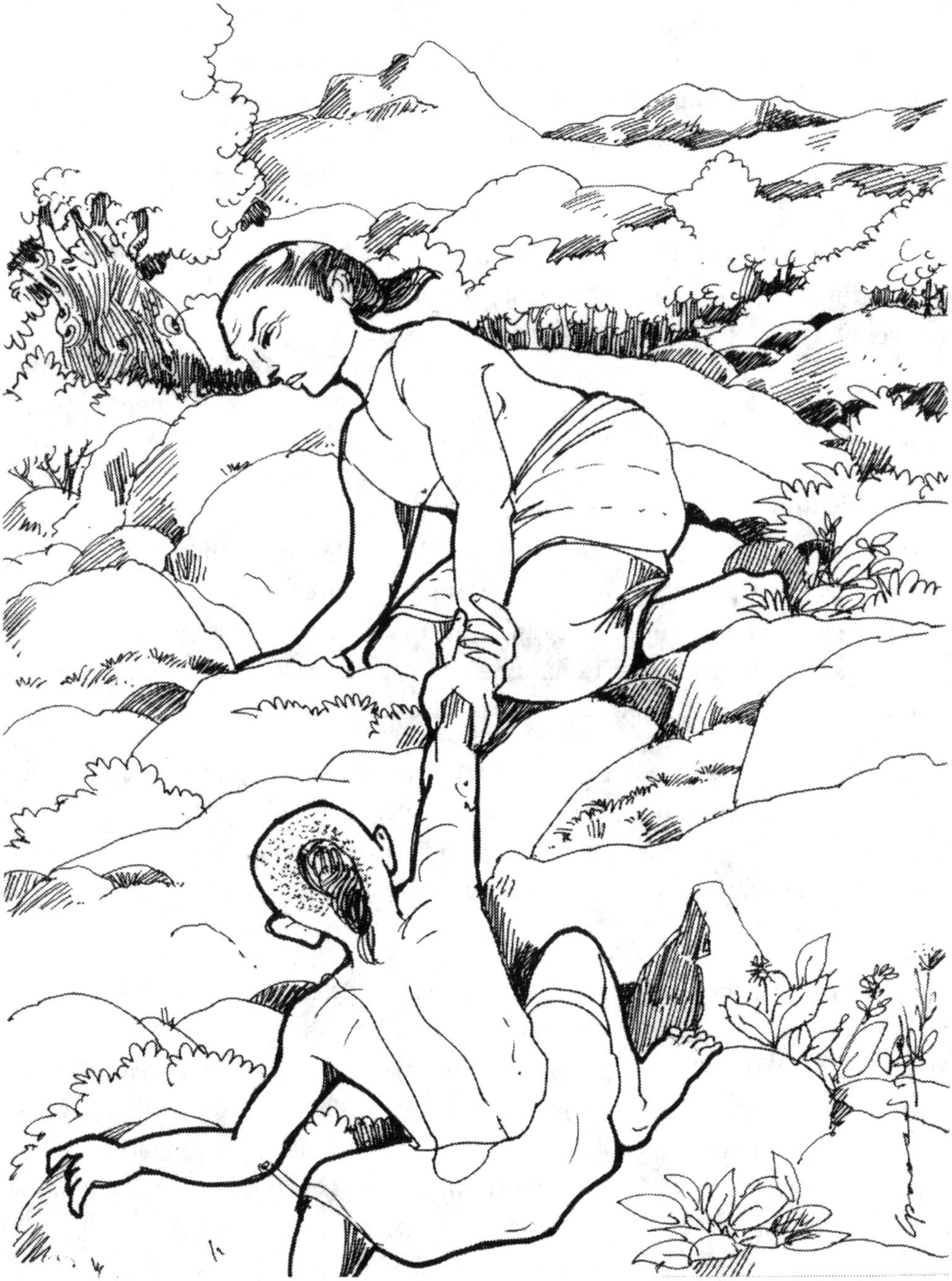

Figure 1: Man in a pit

A man fallen in a pit may climb out on his own, but would welcome the offer of a helping hand. This illustrates a physician's role in treating patients.

Definition

The synonyms of disease included vyādhi, āmaya, gada, ātaṅka, yakṣma, jvara, and vikāra. The "synonymous" status obtained by yakṣma (tuberculosis) and jvara (fever) for disease shows how common and feared these diseases were in ancient India. According to Caraka, the equilibrium of the constituents of the body (dhātus) signifies the healthy condition of an individual and the purpose of his text was to prescribe guidelines for its achievement.[7] Centuries later, Vāgbhaṭa identified the equilibrium of doṣas as the hallmark of good health and their disequilibrium as the marker of disease.[8]

Classifications

Several classifications of diseases were used in Āyurveda based on different criteria.

A classification by Caraka based on causation

Overuse, non-use and misuse of sense objects: This is accepted as an important cause of diseases. An obvious example is gluttony indicative of the over use of taste, starvation implying non-use, and eating junk food pointing to misuse. This example can be multiplied by citing the experience of other senses. According to Caraka, this is a common cause for physical and mental disorders.[9]

External causes: These are beyond the control of human beings, which affect large numbers regardless of their constitutional type, age, and gender. The diseases, injuries, and out breaks would be many. Examples are earthquakes, floods, drought, and destruction of the habitat (janapadodhvamsana).

Prajñāparādha: This term is used by Caraka to indicate a combination of imprudent conduct arising from an error of understanding.[10, 11] There are numerous examples of individuals adopting and persisting with habits which are harmful to them. Many of the current non-communicable diseases such as diabetes, coronary artery disease, and several cancers are preventable by careful attention to diet, physical activity, and avoidance of smoking; but millions are unwilling or unable to follow the sane advice. This is due to prajñāparādha, which is an unfortunate trait of the human condition.

A classification by Suśruta[12]

Suśruta's classification is more compact and widely used. It groups diseases under seven categories (Table 1).

Table 1: Classification of Diseases

Type	Comments
Ādhyātmika	
1. Hereditary (ādibala)	Inherited through defective semen or ovum. E.g.: leprosy, piles
2. Congenital (janmabala)	Present at birth due to the unwholesome conduct of mother during pregnancy; may be dietary indiscretions or neglect of foetal needs. E.g.: lameness, blindness, deaf-mute, etc.
3. Doṣa-induced (doṣabala)	Caused by doṣas which are perturbed by dietary indiscretions, imprudent conduct; perturbations may be located in the stomach or further down in the gut. They may manifest as diseases of the body and mind.
Ādhibhautika	
4. Traumatic (samghātabala)	Due to injuries sustained when the weak is pitted against the strong; may be caused by weapons or by ferocious beasts.
Ādhidaivika	
5. Seasonal (kālabala)	Caused by cold, heat, wind, rains, and other seasonal factors, which may occur in excess or may be too little or out of season.
6. Supernatural (daivabala)	By the wrath of gods, curse of saints and offensive rituals of Atharvaveda. The events may be lightning, those caused by evil spirits, etc. They may be contagious (saṃsargaja) or accidental.
7. Natural (svabhāvabala)	At the root of these disorders are urges such as hunger, thirst, sleep, senile debility, and death (of body tissues); they may be timely or untimely depending on whether they occur in spite of observing the code of good conduct or living in violation of it.

Suśruta added that vāta, pitta, and kapha are the fundamental causes of all diseases. Not only scriptures proclaim, but experience also attests to the fact that perturbation of doṣas leads to disease and their pacification restores normalcy. Diseases in diverse forms and locations are the expressions of diverse and changing combination of doṣas, body constituents (dhātus), and malas; and different sites of the perturbation of doṣas and different precipitating factors (nimitta).

Other classifications: There are several other classifications of diseases such as:

a) Based on bhūtas: āgneya (paittika), saumya (kaphaja), vātika (vātika)

b) Psychologic: rājasa, tāmasa

c) Based on prognosis: curable (sādhya), curable with difficulty (kṛcchra sādhya), asādhya (incurable)

d) Based on clinical findings:
   - Internal (caused by doṣa perturbation)
   - External (caused by spirits including organisms or bhūtas, polluted air, fire, trauma)
   - Psychologic (caused by unfulfilled desires, advent of the undesired)

e) Based on the pathway of disease:[13]
   - Along the surface of the body: skin and rasa dhātu and blood within it Middle layer; location of important organs such as urinary bladder, heart, bone, and joints
   - Deepest layer: this is the gut extending from the oral cavity to the anus

No wonder Caraka remarked that while classifications of diseases may specify a certain number, they may be considered innumerable from various other points of view.[14] As diseases are innumerable and doṣas are limited in number, Caraka favoured a simple classification of diseases based on vāta, pitta, and kapha and two psychic doṣas – rājasa and tāmasa.[15]

Diseases-stages in evolution

It is well known that individuals who have appeared and felt well may suddenly become comatose or die with no prior warning. But, the majority of ailments are preceded by a period of days or even weeks when the individual may feel tired, feverish, have poor appetite and sleep, and experience malaise. This period between the onset of vague symptoms and the appearance of the full-blown picture of a disease was of great interest in Āyurveda. A study of this period, when the disease was incubating and spreading its reach in the body, it was felt, would enable physicians to detect time windows when a therapeutic intervention would be most effective and appropriate.

The progress of imperceptible events in the body during the incubation period could be called disease process or patho-physiology in modern terminology. It begins when a breach in the equilibrium of doṣas and dhātus occurs due to a cause (nidāna) which also perturbs a doṣa, and the perturbed doṣa in turn disturbs a body component (dhātu). The triggering of the disease process calls for three factors – cause, doṣa, and dhātu or dūṣya. The characteristics of vāta, pitta, and kapha, which are described in detail and their relative strengths vis-à-vis the characteristics and strength of the dhātus they assail would largely determine the speed, severity, and course of the diseases process. Other factors, which would influence the disease process are; the drugs administered to the patient, food consumed, season, conduct, and anxious behaviour of the patients.

Though Caraka does refer to disease process in terms of its start with a cause, the unmanifested or partially manifested state (pūrvarūpa), and fully manifested state,[16] a fuller description is given by Suśruta as a six-stage process[17], where each stage is designated as a "kriyākāla." The staging is based on the natural location, perturbation, and subsequent changes taking place in the three doṣas.

The three doṣas have their natural abodes in the body. The natural home of vāta is the pelvis, rectum, and anus. Above this and below, the umbilicus lies the lower gut. Pitta has its abode between the lower gut and stomach. Stomach is the host of kapha. The natural location of the three doṣas are important when the perturbation of doṣas and its progression are being considered as a six-stage process.

1) *Caya (accumulation):* On perturbation by various causes, doṣas accumulate in their respective locations. The patient may feel flatulence, feeling of cold, heaviness of body parts, and lassitude.

2) *Prakopa (perturbation aggravated):* Vāta, pitta, and kapha have many specific factors, which cause perturbation and its progression. For example, vāta is perturbed by violent physical activity, keeping awake at night, suppression of natural physical urges, and cold season; pitta by grief and anger, fasting, sour/salty/hot food, wines, oil and oil cakes, autumn season; kapha by day sleep, sweet/sour/salty/slimy food, incompatible food items, winter season: blood by liquid/greasy food, day sleep, anger, over exposure to sun and seasons, which disturb other doṣas.

   In this stage, patients may complain of pricking pain and gurgling in the abdomen, acid eructation, thirst, loss of appetite, and nausea.

3) *Prasara (spread):* The quantity of perturbed doṣas increases and they begin to flow like "fermented rice water" throughout the body. What drives the fluid is vāyu, which is rājasic and the torrential flow will engulf other doṣas including blood singly or in combination. The result may be the disease affecting the whole body or a part of it. It is possible that perturbed doṣas may remain quiescent in the absence of proper treatment only to flare up on a later date.

   The patient would complain of nausea and borborygmi in vāta perturbation with spread, localised, or generalized burning and eructation in the disturbance and spread of pitta; and loss of appetite, lassitude and vomiting in the disturbance, and spread of kapha.

This stage is an opportunity to treat the condition.

4) *Sthāna* saṃśraya *(localisation of perturbed doṣas):* The perturbed doṣas travel all over the body and find lodgement in different parts or organs such as abdomen, urinary bladder, pelvis, rectum, head and neck, skin, muscle, blood, adipose tissue, bone, extremities or, all over the body. The signs and symptoms of this localisation will be characteristic of the affected body part or organs. For example, the lodgement of perturbed doṣas in the urinary bladder may produce retention of urine, urolithiasis, etc., but the course of the disease may manifest in the features of vāta, pitta, or kapha depending on which doṣa is perturbed.

   This is the prodromal stage when treatment is necessary and justified.

5) *Vy*ādhidarśanam *(manifestation of the disease):* In this stage, the full-blown picture of the disease appears with conspicuous features such as generalised swelling, abscess, cellulitis, high fever, and diarrhoea.

6) *Vraṇa (late manifestations and complications):* Localised diseases may break out into ulcers in a later stage and be accompanied by chronic fever, diarrhoea and other debilitating features. If treatment is not carried out at this late stage, the disease will become incurable.

   Ideally, the disease should be treated at the first stage of accumulation, so that further progress is aborted. As the disease progresses to later stages, the perturbation of doṣas would gain greater strength. During the six stages of the disease process, one severely perturbed doṣa may perturb other doṣas and aggravate the illness. In treating doṣa perturbation under varied conditions, the appropriate policy is to counter the primarily deranged doṣa while taking care that the therapy does not perturb other doṣas. Vāgbhaṭa pointed out that therapeutics which settled one disease and triggered another is a flawed practice of medicine.[18]

Manifestations of doṣa perturbation[19]

Vāta: Among the numerous diseases caused by vāta perturbation, eighty are most important. They are characterised by certain common features, which are expressions of the properties of vāta. The varied manifestations in the vāta affected organs and tissues include divisions, separations, dislocation, attachment, tearing, discomfort, jubilation, thirst, tremors, looseness, pain, movement, roughness, porosity, reddish colour, astringent or absent taste, wasting, numbness, stiffness, limping, and so on.

Pitta: There are forty prominent disorders caused by the perturbation of pitta. Here, again the clinical features owe their manifestation to the specific properties of pitta. The features include heat, sharpness, fluidity, colour except white and red, fishy smell, pungent and sour taste, and mobility. In a pitta affected organ or part, burning, heat, sweat, sloughing, itching, discharge with pitta specific colour, and smell are regularly seen.

Kapha: The prominent disorders caused by the perturbation of kapha are twenty in number. Their characteristic features are oiliness, coldness, whiteness, heaviness, sweetness, immobility, numbness, mucinousness, aggregation, and chronicity.

A thorough familiarity with the clinical features of the perturbation of doṣas is indispensable to make a diagnosis of disorders and a plan for therapy.

Doṣa perturbation in generalised and localised diseases

Vāta, pitta, and kapha permeate the entire body and have the "right of way" to travel through all the body conduits. When not perturbed, they promote the well-being of the individual by enhancing strength, complexion, and cheerfulness; when perturbed, they cause a variety of disorders.[20] Body cannot exist without the three doṣas and blood (a fourth doṣa according to Suśruta).[21]

Though doṣas traverse through all the body conduits from their natural locations, they may produce diseases affecting the entire body or only a part of it. Suśruta likened this to the sky being overcast by dark clouds and the rainfall affecting a vast or a limited area.[22] In the fourth stage of the incubation process of a disease, the perturbed doṣa or doṣas migrate to different parts of the body through the ubiquitous srotas, which are not passive channels but active conduits. They are active in so far as they not only share the colour of the dhātu where they are located but also interact with them as well as the substance including doṣas, which they transport. When a perturbed doṣa localises in the gut, urinary bladder, skin, muscle, blood, head and neck, and other organs and tissues, they may produce local diseases that may be serious such as stone in the bladder and retention of urine or minor lesions such as a boil on the skin. If the perturbed doṣa spreads all over uniformly, the patient would have generalized features such as fever and rigor. It may well be that the localisation of perturbed doṣas moving through the srotas may not be a random event and may be precipitated by a specific vulnerability in the dhātu where the srotas are located.

Disease process and body channels (srotas)

It is well recognised that the incubation period between the breach of a state of sāmya by a cause and the manifestation of a disease is critical, because it is the prologue to serious illness. The patient's symptoms in this period may be vague and what happens inside the body during incubation may not be fully known. In the old far off days when no tests to determine biochemical or immunological changes existed and body imaging was undreamt of, the incubation period carried an element of mystery. Caraka in fact, remarked that a physician who cannot explore the dark interior of the body with the lamp of knowledge and discrimination is incapable of treating patients successfully.[23] The method adopted by ancient physicians to explore the dark interior –unseen and unobservable - was to use their creative imagination and develop a hypothesis of what might be happening inside the body behind the disease phenomena. Indeed, doing great science is rooted in the construction of an imaginative hypothesis and its testing by appropriate experiments.

Āyurveda is replete with examples of hypothesis such as, the decay of the body when rasāyana prevents degenerative changes, and the mechanism of action of pañcakarma in ridding the body of accumulated doṣas. We find the creative imagination at work again in Āyurveda, when it was challenged by the question of what might be happening inside the body during the incubation period of diseases. The stages – kālakriyā – described by Suśruta envisaged events taking place in the vast network of invisible channels inside the body. Caraka was the champion - extraordinary of srotas. According to him, srotas were the active conduits of all dhātus, which are dynamic entities undergoing constant transformation.[24]

Srotas: "Srotas are as many as living beings who do not come into existence or decay in their absence," Caraka said. Srotas are ubiquitous in the body, because they pervade all the seven dhātus. But the terminology of "srotas" continues to be a puzzle as it is regarded synonymous with sirā, dhamanī, rasāyanī, rasavāhini, nāḍī, pattin, mārga, śarīracchidra, saṃvṛta, sthāna, āśaya, and niketa."[25] As they permeate their resident dhātus, any dysfunction of the srotas would inevitably involve the dhātu as well regardless of whether the dhātu is emerging from its predecessor or is matured. The dysfunction of the srotas would also affect its content, which is being transported. The dysfunctional srotas may also affect related or neighbouring srotas. Finally, perturbed vāta, pitta, and kapha could assail the srotas just as they vitiate dhātus. When a disequilibrium of the doṣa occurs due to whatever reason and doṣas get perturbed, their initial accumulation, spread, localisation, and external manifestation would become more understandable when viewed in the context of these events taking place in the srotas. Moreover, the network of srotas permeates all the seven dhātus, sharing their colour and other properties and transporting a variety of substances. In the call for śodhana therapy in serious ailments, we hear of the elimination of perturbed doṣas from the body, which is in fact a mandate to clear the srotas of the obstructing doṣas. This corroborates the statement that "as long as srotas are normal, the body is not inflicted with any disorder."[26]

Srotas are separate from the dhātus where they are located and they transport a variety of substances such as prāṇa (vital breath), water, nutrients, rasa, blood, muscle, adipose tissue, bone, marrow, semen, urine, faeces, and sweat. This list would clarify that the term srotas includes not only minute and countless channels in the solid dhātus such as muscle and bone, but also larger conduits, which transport air, blood, urine, and faeces.

Classification of srotas based on origin: Srotas are classified based on their origin (mūlam), which is used to explain the clinical features which appear when they are vitiated. A few examples of srotas classified on this basis include the following:

Srotas	Origin	Symptoms
Prāṇavāhika	Heart, Trachea	Disordered breathing
Udakavāhika	Palate, Lung (kloma)	Dry tongue, palate, lip, thirst
Annavāhika	Stomach	Loss of appetite; vomiting
Mūtravāhika	Urinary bladder	Urinary obstruction; polyuria
Svedavāhika	Adipose tissue, Hair follicles	Loss of perspiration; excessive perspiration

Caraka Samhita (CS) has also provided a list of factors, which vitiate each of the srotas arising from different origins.[27]

A few examples follow:[28]

Srotas	Vitiating factors
Prāṇavāhika	Wasting, suppression of urges, starvation
Udakavāhika	Heat, fear, āma, suppression of thirst
Annavāhika	Overeating, untimely eating, incompatible food
Mūtravāhika	Suppression of urge for micturition.
Svedavāhika	Excess physical activity; emotional excess

He concluded his exposition on srotas with the statement that "one who knows the body from all aspects and also all about bodily diseases does not get confused in the practice of medicine."[29] This underlines the importance of the study of human body in health and disease.

Terminal illness; signs of impending dissolution

Ancient Āyurvedic texts laid emphasis on the outcome of illness as well as of therapy. This emphasis reached the zenith in its attitude to terminal illness and the extraordinary effort to look for signs in the body and its environment for the dissolution of the body. Three categories of signs were observed which could possibly herald impending death.[30] These were birthmarks, which were empirically associated with premature death and were regarded as fatal signs. The second category of signs was part of the unfavourable course of the disease such as eruptions or rash on the body, bluish discoloration, and so on. The third category of signs was neither congenital nor disease –related but seemed to appear without a cause. This category of signs was the most significant from the point of view of imminent mortality. Based on five senses, many of these signs known as "riṣṭas" are listed below:

Complexion and voice:

- Abnormal – bluish, blackish, white, green – discoloration of body parts, which may be asymmetrical
- Abnormal discoloration of nails, eyes, urine, facces, feet, lips in patients with severe loss of strength
- Sudden feebleness of voice, unclear speech, very different from the usual style
- One half of the face appears oily and wet but the other half is dry.
- Black spots, freckles appear suddenly on the face.
- Muddy coating on teeth, blue lips; rapid emaciation

Smell and Taste:

Just as a flower precedes the appearance of a fruit, riṣṭa was believed to presage death. It was emphasised that a fruit may appear without a preceding flower but "there is no death without riṣṭas."[31] A few examples of riṣṭa concerning the body in disease are given below:

- Fragrance of various forest flowers in bloom emitting from the body;
- Objectionable odour emitting from the body; etc.

When the above smells appear suddenly and without an apparent cause, death will follow within a year. The abnormal taste appearing in the body of a terminal patient may be pleasant or unpleasant. This is inferred by the swarming of lice, stinging insects, flies, and mosquitoes in the body or their fleeing from it.

Touch:

There are signs of imminent death in relation to the sensation of touch.

- Coldness, sweating, loss of pulsations, loss of flesh and blood on the feet, thighs, buttocks, abdomen, sides, back, hands, lips, and forehead. Flaccidity, distorted position of ankle, knee, shoulder, wrist, and several other parts of the body are also fatal signs.
- Laboured or shallow breathing, loss of pulsation in the neck, matted eye lashes, sunken and open eyes, white teeth with gravel, colour blindness of a mongoose, absence of pain on pulling out hairs, blue colour of the nails are also fatal signs.

Fatal signs from patient's sensory experience:

A series of misperceptions where the patient sees lunar/solar eclipse, when it does not exist; or sees invisible objects, while not seeing visible objects are also listed among fatal signs.

The 12 chapters in the Indriya Sthāna of CS are devoted to terminal illness and signs and symptoms of impending death detected by the physician by using his five senses and from the patient's bizarre and morbid experiences, which were believed to precede death. Though the passage of many centuries, revolutionary advances in medical and surgical treatment and significant changes in social customs and beliefs would call for a reappraisal of the fatal signs in the ancient text, the physical and mental status of the dying patient continues to be a topic of profound importance.

References:

1. M S Valiathan. *The Legacy of Caraka*. OrientBlackswan, Chennai 2003. Introduction xlvi-xlvii.
2. *CS Sūtra* 10: 7 - 8
3. *CS Nīdana* 6: 4
4. *CS Nīdana* 6: 6
5. *AH Uttara* 40: 64
6. *AV* 8 (7): 23 – 24. M S Valiathan. Quoted in Page: xviii. *The Legacy of Caraka*. Orient Blackswan, Chennai 2003.
7. *CS Sūtra* 1: 53 – 55
8. *AH Sūtra* 12: 32 - 33
9. *CS Sūtra* 1: 54
10. *CS Vimāna* 6: 6

11. *CS* Śārīra 1: 102 - 108
12. *SS Sūtra* 24: 4 – 8
13. *CS Sūtra* 11: 48
14. *CS Vimāna* 6: 3
15. *CS Vimāna* 6: 5
16. *CS Nīdana* 1: 6 - 11
17. *SS Sūtra* 21: 6 – 35
18. *AH Sūtra* 13: 16
19. *CS Sūtra* 20: 10 - 18
20. *CS Sūtra* 20: 9 - 10
21. *SS Sūtra* 21: 3
22. *SS Sūtra* 21: 30
23. *CS Vimāna* 4: 12
24. *CS Vimāna* 5: 3 - 4
25. *CS Vimāna* 5: 9
26. *CS* Vimāna 5: 7
27. *CS* Vimāna 5: 10 - 22
28. *CS* Vimāna 5: 10 – 22
29. *CS* Vimāna 5: 31
30. *CS* Indriya 1: 5
31. *CS* Indriya 2: 4 - 5

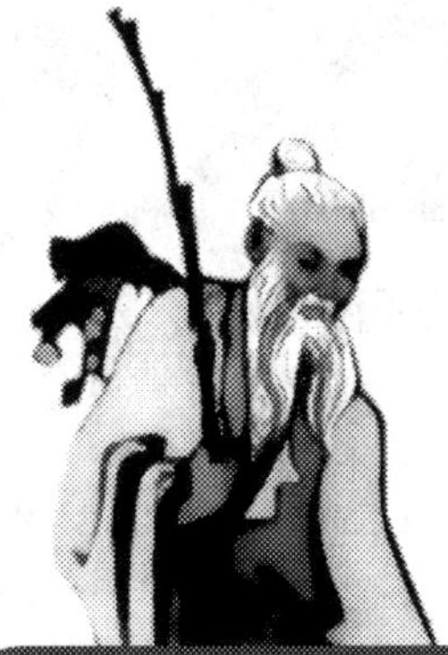

CHAPTER 7

Food and Drinks

Āyurveda attached the highest importance to food and drinks in the maintenance of good health (svasthavṛtta) and in the genesis and treatment of diseases (āturavṛtta). One of the major discussions in CS which drew the vigorous participation of many sages was based on a question by Vāmaka, King of Kāśī, "Do the humans and their diseases trace back their origins to the same source?"[1] The sage participants could not agree on the identification of a single source of health and disease in individuals and each speaker argued for his candidate source which included self, mind, rasa – a product of digestion and forerunner of dhātus, six dhātus upheld by Sāṅkhya philosophers, parents, karma, nature, and even Prajāpati. However, each point of view was refuted in the discussion and Ācārya Punarvasu who chaired the meeting brought it to a close by drawing everyone's attention to the futility of polemics and the fallacy of parading points of view as facts. He was candid in stating that wholesome food promotes the growth of an individual and unwholesome food is the cause of disorders.[2] Wholesome food is that food which maintains the equilibrium of dhātus and restores equilibrium when it is perturbed. He explained to the assembly that those who understand dietetics (āhāratatva) which covers the properties, composition, effect, and other factors such as the quantity of food would have no difficulty in giving suitable instructions on food and drinks to the community of physicians. The Ācārya himself gave an elaborate exposition on the classifications of food, wholesome and unwholesome food, food as medication and the role of dietary regimen or, pathya in therapy.

Dietetics in the training of physicians: Dietetics was not only a major topic for discussions in the Gurukulas under the chairmanship of the preceptor, but was also for discourses by the preceptor. Furthermore, the students who lived with the preceptor and his family served as apprentices and had ample opportunities to learn the dietetic practices in Āyurveda and acquire manual skills. The duties of the in-house students included the harvest of firewood for the kitchen, collecting medicinal plants, assisting the cooks for preparing meals for the preceptor and his extended family of pupils, and for the preparation of formulations for patients. As the students had to accompany the preceptor for domiciliary visits and examination of patients, spend hours memorizing and learning authoritative texts and taking part in discussions, their life of six or seven years in the Gurukula was hard. However, they were assured of high quality training with equal attention to the acquisition of knowledge and skills and the development of flawless conduct.

In regard to food and drinks, the students would learn all about eatables derived from vegetable and animal sources, their grouping in terms of physical properties such as heavy/light into 20 categories and their effects which may be wholesome or unwholesome. They would know the wholesome and unwholesome items among cereals, pulses, salts, waters, terrestrial, and aquatic animals and birds. It was obligatory for them to learn 152 items covering diet, drugs, and rules of conduct in relation to maintaining health and treating diseases.[3] The extraordinary attention paid to the materials and methods in preparing food and formulations is indicated by Vāgbhaṭa in his description of herbal drugs.[4] Though his primary focus was on herbal drugs, he gave detailed directions on the cooking of fat and assessing properly cooked fat. He also classified cooking based on the physical properties of the end product as soft (manda), medium (chikkaṇa), and hard (kharacikkaṇa). The quantities of various items used in cooking were also specified. The ancient descriptions should leave us in no doubt that a graduate emerging from the Gurukulas on the completion of training would be a competent dietician, cook, and supervisor of a kitchen. He would also know a good deal about incompatible foods, food poisoning, and how to protect the King from deliberate poisoning by enemies. Physicians aspired to be appointed as royal physicians, which entitled them to escort the Kings during military campaigns, have a tent next to the King's and ensure the safety of the raw and cooked food served to the King in his meals.[5]

Patient's diet: Food and drinks are among the longest and most detailed chapters in CS and SS. Caraka says, "food and drinks with agreeable smell, taste, and touch and having been taken as per prescribed method provides vitality and strength. This has been observed by experts directly. The fire (agni) which sustains life within the body cannot burn in the absence of its fuel (food and drinks)."[6] If food and drinks are ill chosen, ill prepared or ill served, the consequences will be harmful.

As food and drinks cover a wide range of products of vegetables, animal, and mineral origin it is necessary to classify them for easier understanding.

General Classification:

1. Śūkadhānya (grains with husk)
2. Śamīdhānya (pulses)
3. Māṃsa (meats)
4. Śāka (vegetables)
5. Phala (fruits)
6. Harita (greens)
7. Madya (alcoholic drinks)
8. Jala (water)
9. Gorasa (milk and milk products)
10. Ikṣu (sugarcane products)

Cooked preparations (kṛtānnas) and food additives (āhārayogī) are listed separately (Table 1-12) as they are not primary categories of food and drinks.

The sub-classifications of the ten categories are given in Tables 1–11.

Table 1: Grains (śūkadhānyas**)***[, 7]

Sl No	Names	Qualities	Other effects in the body
1	Śālī varieties (rice)	Cold, sweet, lubricant	Promotes bulk, semen; Promotes output of urine
2	Ṣāṣṭikā varieties (rice)	Cold, lubricant, sweet, stable	Promotes bulk, semen; Promotes output of urine
3	Vrīhi (rice)	Sweet, heavy	Promotes output of urine and faeces
4	Śyāmāka (rice)	Astringent, sweet, light, cold	Constipating
5	Hastiśyāmāka family (rice)	Astringent, sweet, light, cold	Constipating
6	Yava (barley)	Rough, cold, non-heavy, sweet, astringent	Bulky stools, easy flatus; promotes stability
7	Veṇuyava (Bamboo seeds)	Rough, astringent, sweet	Strengthening; good for obesity, helminthiasis and poisoning
8	Godhūma (wheat)	Sweet, cold, heavy, lubricant, uniting	Promotes corpulence
9	Nāndīmukhī, Madhulī (wheat varieties)	Sweet, lubricant, cold	-

*Cereals are ideal for use when a year old. The old is rough, the new is heavy. The crop, which matures, is lighter in quality.

Table 2: Pulses (śamidhānya)*,8

Sl No	Names	Qualities	Other effects in the body
1	Mudga (green gram)	Astringent, sweet, rough, cold, light, clear, kaṭu vipāka; Best among pulses	
2	Māṣa (black gram)	Lubricant, hot, sweet, heavy	Aphrodisiac, strengthening, produces bulky stools
3	Rājamāṣa (red kidney beans)	Sweet, rough, astringent, clear, heavy	Relieves burning stomach and disorders of semen: laxative
4	Kulattha (horse gram)	Hot, astringent, āmlapāka	Constipating: good for cough, dyspnea, hiccup, and piles
5	Makuṣṭhaka	Sweet, madhurapāka rough, cold	Beneficial in fever, internal bleeding
6	Caṇaka (gram), Masūra (lentil), khaṇḍikā, hareṇu (Peas)	Light, cold, sweet, astringent, rough	Masūra is constipating
7	Tila (sesamum)	Lubricant, hot, sweet bitter, astringent, pungent	Good for skin, hair, body strength
8	Śimbī	Rough, astringent	Digests with wind formation; non-aphrodisiac, not good for eye

* Pulses are ideal for use when a year old. The old is rough, the new is heavy. When dehusked and fried, pulses are digested readily.

Table 3: Meats (māṃsa) *,9

Sl No	Names	Qualities	Other effects in the body
1	Animals, which grab prey (prasahā). E.g.: cow, ass, camel, lion, bear, dog, tiger, cat, mouse, crow, vulture, etc.	Heavy, hot, sweet	Good for phthisis; beneficial in treating unripe and loose stools; strengthens the body
2	Animals living in burrows/ tunnels (bhūmiśaya). E.g.: Python, frog, iguana, mongoose	Madhura vipāka, kaṣāya and kaṭu in rasa (iguana)	Useful for the strong with good digestive power and physical activity in general. Bulk promoting and tonic (iguana)

Sl No	Names	Qualities	Other effects in the body
3	Animals living in wet -land. (ānupamṛga). E.g.: boar, yak, pig, rhinoceros, cow, buffalo, elephant, deer	Heavy, hot, sweet Lubricant, heavy (pork) Lubricant, hot, sweet, heavy (buffalo meat)	Appropriate for those with high level of physical activity and digestion. Obstructs channels, strengthening, promoting, improves complexion (rhinoceros). Bulk promoting, aphrodisiac, improves strength, appetite, sweating (pork). Good for chronic cold, recurrent fever, dry cough, wasting, excessive digestive agni (beef), builds bulk, firmness: improves morale and sleep (buffalo meat)
4	Animals living in water (vāriśaya). E.g.: Tortoise, crab, fish, whale, oyster, crocodile, etc.	Heavy, hot, sweet, lubricant (fish)	Promotes bulk; aphrodisiac, has many defects (fish), good for complexion, improves vision, intellect; destroys phthisis (tortoise)
5	Animals moving on water (vāricārī). E.g.: swan, crane, kāraṇḍava, kadamba, utkrośa, jalakukkuṭī, nandimukhī, cakravāka, etc.	Heavy, hot, sweet	Appropriate for those with high level of physical activity and strong digestion
6	Animals in forests (jāṅgalamṛga). E.g.: Deer, śarabha, hare, eṇa, śambara, kālapucchaka, etc.	Astringent, non-slippery, rough, cold, light, kaṭuvipāka (hare), madhuravipāka, light, cold (eṇa)	Diminishes urinary output, constipating
7	Birds which scatter grain while eating (Lāvādyas). E.g.: common quail, kapiñjala, cakora, kukkubha, etc.	Light, cold, sweet, astringent	Pacifies sannipāta where pitta is dominant and vāta is moderate
8	Birds of the poultry category (vartakādi). E.g.: bustard, peacock, partridge, cock, kaṅka, indrābhā, etc.	Lubricant, hot (cock) Heavy, hot, sweet (partridge)	Improves vision, hearing, intellect, agni, complexion, voice; builds muscle and semen Builds bulk, improves voice, evokes sweating (cock)
9	Birds which eat while striking (pratuda). E.g.: Śatapatrā, kokilā, kapota, śuka, sāraṅga, caṭaka, etc.	Astringent, non-slippery, cold, madhura vipāka (domestic pigeon) Astringent, sour, pungent, cold (parrot), light sweet, lubricant (caṭaka)	Controls internal bleeding (domestic pigeon). Useful in phthisis, appetite; constipating (parrot); Promotes strength and semen (caṭaka)

* Meat of animals which died naturally, killed by poisons or by snakes, tigers, etc., should be discarded; so also, that of too fat, too old, too young, and emaciated. Meat soup is a superior tonic for those with phthisis, emaciation, and other serious ailments.

Table 4: Vegetables (śāka)*, 10

Sl No	Names	Qualities	Other effects in the body
1	Pāṭhā (Kucēlā), kāsamarda, śatī, vāstuka, etc.		Constipating except vāstuka which is laxative
2	Kākamācī	Not too hot or too cold	Aphrodisiac, rasāyana, purgative, anti-leprotic
3	Rājakṣavaka	Light	Constipating: beneficial for piles
4	Kālaśāka	Pungent, light, hot, rough	Improves appetite, good for swellings: antidote to poisons
5	Amlacāṅgērī	Uṣṇavīrya	Appetiser, constipating: beneficial in piles
6	Upodikā	Madhura rasa, lubricant, cold	Purgative, aphrodisiac, anti-narcotic
7	Taṇḍulīya	Rough, cold, madhura rasa	Beneficial in narcosis, poisoning, internal bleeding
8	Maṇḍūkaparṇī, kucelā, bākucī, kembuka, kalāya, nimba, etc.	Śītavīrya, kaṭu vipāka kapha	All are bitter
9	Kuṭumbaka, karbudāra, niṣpāva, kovidāra, kumārajīva, cakramarda, kūśmāṇḍaka, triparṇī, etc.	Heavy, rough, madhura, śītavīrya	Produce abdominal distension during digestion: purgative effect
10	Flowers of śaṇa, kovidāra, etc.	Check flow through channels	Useful in internal bleeding channels
11	Tender leaves of udumbara, aśvattha, lotus, etc.	Astringent, cold, checks flow through channels	Beneficial in pittaja diarrhoea
12	Vatsādanī, gandīra, citraka Śreyasī, bilvaparṇī, bilva leaves	-	
13	Bhandī, śatāvarī, balā, jīvantī, etc.	-	
14	Lāṅgalikā, eraṇḍa	Light, bitter	Purgative
15	Tila, Vētasa	Pungent, bitter, sour	Purgative
16	Kusumbhā	Rough, sour, hot	-
17	Trapusā, ervāruka	Sweet, heavy, cold, rough	Improves urine output; ripe fruit relieves burning sensation, thirst, fatigue

Sl No	Names	Qualities	Other effects in the body
18	Alābu	Rough, cold, heavy	Purgative
19	Ripe fruit of kūśmāṇḍa	Sweet, sour, light alkaline	Diuretic, laxative
20	Kelūṭa, kadamba, etc.	Non-slippery, heavy, cold	Block body channels
21	Utpala varieties	Astringent	Beneficial in internal bleeding
22	Tālapralambha	-	Beneficial in wounds and chest pain
23	Tarūṭa, lotus root and stem, krauñcādana, etc.	Heavy, obstructing, cold	
24	Lotus seeds	Madhura in rasa and vipāka, astringent	Beneficial in internal bleeding
25	Muñjātaka	Cold, heavy, lubricant, sweet	Promotes bulk and strength; aphrodisiac
26	Vidārīkaṇḍa	Sweet and cold	Rasāyana; promotes bulk and strength; beneficial for throat; aphrodisiac
27	Amlīkā tuber	Light, not very hot.	Beneficial in treating unripe and loose stools; piles; alcoholism; constipating
28	Mustard	-	Constipating; diminishes urinary output
29	Mushroom varieties	Cold, sweet, and heavy	Causes rhinitis

* Vegetables contaminated by insects; damaged by wind, sun; old and unseasonal; uncooked in fat and not cleansed should be discarded.

Table 5: Fruits (Phala)*, [11]

Sl No	Names	Qualities	Other effects in the body
1	Grapes	Sweet, cold, lubricant	Relieves fever, dyspnea, thirst, internal bleeding, wasting, hoarse voice, alcoholism, dryness of mouth, cough; bulk promoting; aphrodisiac
2	Āmrāta	Sweet, heavy, slightly lubricant, cold	Promotes bulk; tonic; improves digestion but with distension; aphrodisiac
3	Tāla, nārīkela fruits	Lubricant, cold, sweet	Promotes bulk, tonic
4	Bhavya (kāśmarya very similar)	Sweet, sour, astringent, heavy, cold	Cleanses mouth; constipating

Sl No	Names	Qualities	Other effects in the body
5	Sour fruits. E.g.: parūṣaka, grapes, jujube, etc.	-	-
6	Parāvāta (two types)	Heavy	Reduces excessive digestive agni and appetite
7	Taṅka	Astringent, sweet, heavy, cold	-
8	Kapittha (unripe) (ripe)	-Sweet, sour, astringent, heavy	Constipating; irritates throat; counters poisonsFragrance adds to taste, counters poison, constipating
9	Bilva (unripe) (ripe)	Lubricant, hot sharp-	Improves appetitePoorly digested: flatulent
10	Āmra (unripe) (ripe)	-	Causes internal bleedingPromotes strength, semen and develops muscles
11	Jambū	Astringent, sweet, heavy, cold	Flatulent; constipating
12	Jujube(dried)	Sweet, lubricantSweet, lubricant	Purgative
13	Śimbītakā	Sweet, astringent, cold	Constipating
14	Gāṅgerukī, karīra, bimbī, etc.	Sweet, astringent, cold	-
15	Panasa, moca, rājādana (ripe)	Sweet, astringent, lubricant, cold, heavy	-
16	Lavalī	Astringent, non-slippery, fragrant	Useful as condiment
17	Nīpa, pīlu, ketakī	-	Counter poisons: anti-toxic
18	Iṅgudī	Bitter, sweet, lubricant, hot	-
19	Tinḍuka	Astringent, sweet, light	-
20	Āmalaka	All rasas present except salt; rough, sweet, astringent, sour	-
21	Bibhītaka	-	Good for disorders of rasa, blood, muscle and fat; improves voice, pittaja diseases, and copious sputum
22	Dāḍima	Sour, astringent, sweet, lubricant	Controls diarrhoea
23	Vṛkṣāmḷa (ripe tamarind has a similar effect)	Rough, hot	Controls diarrhoea

Sl No	Names	Qualities	Other effects in the body
24	Amḷavetasa	Rough, hot	Beneficial in bowel disorders, loss of appetite, hiccup, alcoholism, cough and dyspnea, and vāta and kapha disorders
25	Karcūra (without skin)	-	Improves appetite; beneficial in dyspnea, hiccup and piles
26	Nāgaraṅga	Sweet, mildly sour; heavy	Improves appetite; difficult to digest
27	Vātāma, abhiṣuka, etc.(priyāla is similar except it is not hot)	Heavy, hot, lubricant, sweet	Promotes bulk; aphrodisiac
28	Śļeṣmātaka	Sweet, cold	
29	Aṅkoṭa	Heavy	Diminishes digestive agni: causes abdominal distension
30	Karañja	-	Flatulent
31	Āmṛātaka, dantaśatha, etc. (sour)	-	Causes internal bleeding
32	Vārtāka	Pungent, bitter	Improves appetite
33	Ākṣikī	Sour	-
34	Aśvattha, uḍumbara, etc.	Astringent, sweet, sour, heavy	-
35	Bhallātaka (stone of fruit) (flesh)	Fiery, sweet, cold	

*Old, rotten, and unripe fruits; those damaged by insects, animals, snow, and sun; or grown in unnatural place and wrong season are unfit to eat.

Table 6: Greens (harita)*, 12

Sl No	Names	Qualities	Other effects in the body
1	Ādraka (ginger)		Improves appetite; aphrodisiac; Relieves constipation
2	Jambīra	Relieves vāta and kapha	Improves appetite, fragrant, cleans mouths, digestive; good for treating worms; Irritant
3	Mūlaka (Radish) (Old) (Fried in fat) (Dried)		 Relieves three doṣas Relieves vāta Relieves vāta and kapha
4	Surasā	Perturbs pitta Relieves kapha and vāta	Removes cough, foul smell, shortness of breath, and pain on the sides of the trunk

Sl No	Names	Qualities	Other effects in the body
5	Yavānī, śigru, etc.	Perturbs pitta	Juice is pleasing
6	Gandīra, jalapippalī, etc.	Hot, pungent, rough	
7	Bhūstṛṇa	Pungent, hot, rough	Cleans mouth, harmful to sexual potency
8	Dhānyaka; ajagandhā, etc.	Not very pungent	Appetising, fragrant
9	Gṛñjanaka	Beneficial in vāta and kapha disorders	Constipating, irritant; good for piles: useful in fomentation and in the diet for those without pittaja disorders irritant
10	Palāṇḍu	Heavy	Useful in diet; promotes strength; aphrodisiac; appetising
11	Laśuna	Lubricant, hot, pungent, heavy	Good for treating worms, leprosy, leucoderma, gaseous abdominal swelling; aphrodisiac

* Individual properties are superseded by the steps in cooking and processing.

Table 7: Alcoholic drinks (madya)[13]

Sl No	Names	Qualities	Other effects in the body
1	Surā	Relieves vāta	Useful for treating emaciation, gaseous abdominal swelling, urinary obstruction, insufficient lactation, piles
2	Madirā	Relieves vāta	Useful for treating hiccup, dyspnea, cough, vomiting, difficult defecation, constipation
3	Jagalā	Rough, hot	Beneficial for colic, dysentery, borborygmi, piles; constipating
4	Ariṣṭa	Relieves kapha disorders	Useful for treating phthisis, piles, loss of appetite, fever, anaemia, abdominal swelling
5	Śarkarā		Tasty, intoxicant, fragrant, improves digestion; relieves disorders of urinary bladder
6	Pakvarasa	Relieves kapha disorders	Improves appetite, complexion, useful in treating phthisis, swelling, piles
7	Śītārasikā		Improves digestion, voice and complexion; beneficial in swelling, abdominal disorders, piles; useful for slimming
8	Gauḍa		Eases passage of flatus and faeces; improves appetite
9	Akṣikī		Improves appetite; good for treating anaemia and wounds

Sl No	Names	Qualities	Other effects in the body
10	Surāsava	Relieves vāta	Strong intoxicant; tasty
11	Madhvāsava	Sharp	Expectorant
12	Maireya	Sweet and heavy	
13	Āsava of grapes, sugar cane juice with dhātakī flowers	Rough, not very hot	Expectorant
14	Madhu	Light	Relieves constipation, improves appetite effect on vāta
15	Surā with maṇḍa of barley gruel (upper clear layer)	Rough, hot	Perturbs vāta and pitta
16	Madhūlikā	Heavy	Produces flatulence during digestion
17	Sauravīraka and tuṣōdaka		Improve appetite and digestion; beneficial for abdominal swelling, piles, helmithiasis and heart disorders
18	Sour vinegar; (external application)		Relieves fever and burning sensation (internal use)
19	Fresh wine; Old wine	Heavy;Light	Tasty, improves appetite, opens body channels

Table 8: Milk and Dairy products (Gorasa)[14]

Sl No	Names	Qualities	Other effects in the body
1	Cow's milk	Sweet, cold, soft, lubricant, viscous, smooth, slippery, heavy, slow and pleasant	Best among rasāyanas: enhances ojas
2	Buffalo's milk	Heavier and colder than cow's milk; rich in fat	Good for sleeplessness and for those with powerful digestion
3	Camel's milk	Rough, hot, mildly, saltish, light	Useful for treating constipation, worms, abdominal disorders, piles, and swelling
4	Mare's, ass's milk (one hoofed animals)	Hot, saltish, rough, light	Builds strength, relieves vāta disorders of extremities

Sl No	Names	Qualities	Other effects in the body
5	Goat's milk	Astringent, sweet, cold, light	Constipating; beneficial for internal bleeding, diarrhoea, wasting, cough and fever
6	Sheep's milk	Hot	Causes hiccup, shortness of breath
7	Elephant's Milk	Heavy, builds strength	Stabilises body
8	Human milk	Lubricant	Vitalising; builds strength and revives life energy; used as local application in nose and eye for treating bleeding and pain, respectively
9	Curd	Lubricant, hot, āmlapāka	Improves appetite: builds strength; indicative of good fortune; aphrodisiac; beneficial in nasal diseases, diarrhoea, fevers, loss of appetite, difficult urination and emaciation. To be discarded in autumn, summer and spring
10	Maṇḍaka (not fully matured curd)	Perturbs three doṣas; mature curd relives vāta	Supernatant layer formed on milk promotes semen: diluted curd opens body channels
11	Buttermilk	-	Useful in the treatment of piles, abdominal disorders, urinary obstruction, swelling, poor appetite and excess disorders fat in the body and poisoning
12	Fresh butter	-	Improves appetite: induces constipation; improves abdominal disorders, piles, poor appetite, facial paralysis
13	Ghee (cow's)	Cold, sweet, madhura-vipāka	Best of all fats: thousands of actions: improves intelligence, semen, ojas, kapha and medas; useful in treating poisoning, insanity, fever, phthisis; old cow's ghee for intoxication, seizures, phthisis, pain in the ear and head, pain in the female genitalia.
14	Milk varieties and preparations. E.g.: colostrum, condensed milk, etc.	Heavy	Saturating; promotes bulk; appropriate for those with excellent digestion, poor sleep: aphrodisiac

Table 9: Sugarcane Products (ikṣu)[15]

Sl No	Names	Qualities	Other effects in the body
1	Sugarcane juice	Cold, lubricant, sweet	Laxative, promotes bulk; causes acidity (with machine- pressed juice)
2	Jaggery	-	Builds blood, marrow, fat muscle: encourages worms
3	Sugar (from Jaggery) (from yāsa) (from honey)	Cold, sweet, lubricant. Astringent, sweet, cold, mildly bitter Rough	All sugars good for thirst, internal bleeding, and heartburn Beneficial for the injured; aphrodisiac Anti-emetic, anti-diarrheal, and expectorant
4	Honey (from mākṣika) (from bhramara) (from Kṣaudra) (from pauttika)	Oil like in colour; Heaviest, white; Brownish colour; Ghee like colour; All are cold, rough, sweet, heavy, astringent	Mākṣika best among honeys. All honeys promote union and expectoration; Forbidden for those suffering from heat

Table 10: Dietary preparations (kṛtānna)[16]

Sl No	Names	Qualities	Other effects in the body
1	Gruel (thin, peya) (thick, vilepikā) (water from gruel Maṇḍa) Water from gruel of fried paddy	Light Light Light	Improves appetite, bowel movement, relieves hunger and thirst, fever and bowel disorders, induces sweat Constipating, agreeable, filling Improves appetite, induces sweat, softens channels; useful in reducing therapy Relieves thirst, diarrhoea; improves appetite; agreeable; beneficial in fainting and heartburn Beneficial for women, children, weak persons
2	Boiled rice	Well-cooked is light;Not well cooked is heavy	Boiled rice prepared with meat, green/black gram, sesamum, oil, ghee, marrow, fruits, etc., builds strength and bulk
3	Boiled rice and spiced grains	Heavy, rough	Induces purgation
4	Flour of roasted grains	Rough	Improves digestion: produces bulky stools; promotes strength quickly in liquid form-that from śāl rice is especially beneficial
5	Barley preparations	-	Good for treating cold and cough, throat diseases and diabetes

Sl No	Names	Qualities	Other effects in the body
6	Fried grain preparations	Heavy	Reducing corpulence; digests with difficulty; Rice flour heaviest
7	Food items cooked with additives like fruits, meat, fat, sesamum paste, and honey	Heavy	Promotes bulk and strength; aphrodisiac
8	Food items prepared with jaggery, milk, honey, and sugar	Very heavy	Promotes strength; aphrodisiac
9	Flattened rice	Heavy	Promotes health
10	Wheat preparations with/in fatWheat preparations made with fried grains, parpaṭa, etc.	Heavy saturatingLight	Aphrodisiac
11	Preparations of pulses	Rough, cold	To be taken in small quantity with spices, fat, etc.
12	Rasālā	Lubricant, tasty	Promotes bulk, strength; aphrodisiac
13	Curd with jaggery	Lubricant	Saturating
14	Syrups, E.g.: dates, grapes, jujube, etc.	Heavy	Flatulent; Action may vary depending on ingredients and their quantities
15	Preparation of sago and ṣāḍava	Pungent, sour, sweet, salty, light	Appetising, palatable
16	Cream–like preparations of āmalaka, etc.	Sweet, heavy, lubricant	Appetising, promotes corpulence
17	Sūkta (a form of vinegar)		Properties and actions depend on the source such as tubers, roots, fruits, etc.
18	Śindākī (a fermented drink)	Light	Improves appetite

Table 11: Food additives (āhāra yogī)[17]

Sl No	Names	Qualities	Other effects in the body
1	Sesamum oil	Sweet, astringent, hot	Best among vāta relieving agents. Constipating; reduces urine output; promotes strength, intellect; by processing with medicinal plants, counters all diseases
2	Castor oil	Sweet, heavy	Useful in treating abdominal swelling, chronic fever, and heart disease
3	Mustard oil	Pungent, hot	Relieves itching and skin rash; reduces semen

Sl No	Names	Qualities	Other effects in the body
4	Prīyāla oil	Sweet, heavy, hot	Because of hotness, not advisable in vāta and pitta disorders
5	Linseed oil	Sweet, sour, kaṭu vipāka, uṣṇa vīrya	
6	Kusumbha oil	Hot, heavy, kaṭu vipāka	Causes heart burn
7	Marrow and animal fat	Sweet; hot or cold according to the habitat aphrodisiac of animals	Builds bulk and strength
8	Dry ginger	Slightly lubricant, hot, madhura vipāka	Improves appetite; aphrodisiac
9	Long pepper (green) (dry)	Sweet, heavy, lubricant. Pungent, hot	Aphrodisiac
10	Black pepper	Light, not very hot	Improves appetite
11	Asafoetida (Hiṅgu)	Pungent, hot, light	Digestive; relieves spasm; binds bowels; appetising
12	Rock salt	Slightly sweet	Best among salts; improves appetite, vision; aphrodisiac
13	Sauvarcalā salt	Hot, light, fragrant	Improves appetite: laxative
14	Biḍa salt	Sharp, hot, quickly absorbed	Appetiser, relieves colic; expels wind
15	Audbhida salt	Pungent, bitter, sharp	Irritant
16	Black salt	All the properties of sauvarcalā except fragrance	
17	Sāmudra salt	Mildly sweet	
18	Yāvaśūka (alkali obtained from barley husk)	Sharp, hot, rough	Beneficial for treating heart disease, pallor, abdominal swelling, constipation, piles, throat complaints
19	Kāravī, Kuñcikā, ajāji, etc.		Improves appetite, remove foul smell

Tables 1 to 11, bear testimony to the richness, variety and rational basis of classifying food and drinks in Āyurveda. This classification of Caraka is followed with some variations in SS. The time for harvesting grains, characterization of birds, animals and fish, caution on pollution, and many other details in the classification highlight the importance attached to food and drinks in Āyurveda. It is noteworthy that an effort was made in correlating each food item with its effect on the doṣas and also other effects on the body. This is crucial because the effects on doṣas could become a cause for their perturbation leading to disequilibrium and disease; additionally, the information on the cause for doṣa perturbation would arm the physician with cues to a find a remedy, which could neutralise the causative factor.

Modern dietetics lays stress on the primary human requirements of carbohydrates, protein, fat and accessory requirements of vitamins, and shadow nutrients. The Tables 1 to 11 from CS address these requirements adequately and exhibit an admirable understanding of the ecology, farming practices, and food habits of the people in the "old, far-off days" in north-west India.

In the discussion on the qualities of food, these are frequent references to heaviness and lightness especially with reference to animal products. Heaviness and lightness of food articles are important to delicate, weak, or sick individuals whose digestive power may be sub-normal, but they may not be relevant to a strong, active individual who toils all day.[18] The determinants of heaviness and lightness are many and some examples are habitat of the animal, part of the animal, gender, size, cooking procedure, additives used in cooking, and quantity consumed. These discussions show an excellent understanding of animal sciences and the transformative effect of cooking on food.

With reference to quantity, "whatever quantity of food taken gets digested in time without disturbing normalcy should be regarded as the measure of proper quantity"[19] for an individual. According to Vāgbhaṭa, "while eating a meal, half the stomach should be filled by solids, a quarter by liquids, and a quarter left for free air flow."[20] "Heavy substances" may behave as if they are "light" when consumed in small quantities, whereas "light" items may become "heavy" when eaten in large quantities. This contrasting action is accounted by the digestive fire on which the strength, health, life span, and vital breath depend. Consuming food, Caraka stressed, was not only to meet a biological necessity, but also for enjoyment. He urged that food should be looked upon as an offering to the digestive fire, giving it the same significance as when oblations are offered to the sacrificial fire. According to him, Vedic rituals for attaining heaven are no less dependent on food than working for a living.[21]

Etiquette for Dining: Suśruta had specified that kitchen where food is prepared should be spacious and clean, and cooks and those who served food should be trust-worthy individuals. The dining room should be private and adorned with flowers. The food should be of high quality and enjoyable. Meal should be served only after sanctified water against toxins had been sprinkled on it and auspicious hymns had been chanted.[22]

The diner should occupy an elevated and comfortable seat, be relaxed and looking forward to the meal. The wise individual would eat when he is hungry and enjoy light, oily, largely liquid, and agreeable food in reasonable quantity. He should neither spend too much time over a meal nor rush through it. The general convention is to serve sweet items first, move on to sour and salty in the middle course, and leave the other rasas to the last part. Fruits such as pomegranate, stem and root of lotus, tubers, and sugar cane are recommended for starters. Āmalaka fruit is welcome at any stage.

The elaborate protocol for dining is illustrated by Table 12, which lists the containers to be used for serving various items during a meal.[23]

Table 12:

Item	Served in/on	Comments
Ghee	Iron vessel	
Gruel	Silver vessel	
Fruits and other hard articles	Leaves	
Dried/oily articles	Golden vessel	
Liquids (meat drink), juices, etc.	Silver vessel	
Buttermilk, khaḍa, vegetable soup	Stone vessel	
Boiled and cooled water to drink	Copper vessel	
Syrup/wine	Earthenware	
Rāga, ṣāḍava, saṭṭaka	Glass and quartz containers adorned with vaiḍūrya	
Rice, pulse with lickable items	Large, attractive dish	Cook to serve on a large, handsome plate in front of the patient/person
Fruits, hard and dried items	-	Served on the plate to the right-hand side of the diner
Liquids, juices, syrup, soups, etc.	-	Served on the plate to the left-hand side of the diner
Jaggery, rāga, ṣāḍava, saṭṭaka	-	Served in the middle of the plate between the above two

Guidelines were given for the appropriate timing of meals in winter and summer, and during day and night. Rinsing the mouth, cleaning the tongue and removing food particles from between teeth were recommended after a meal. Eating unclean, left over, stale, and food cooked many hours earlier was forbidden. Detailed instructions were given for one's conduct after meals in relation to food intake, sleep, and exercise. An important guideline was never to eat a second meal before the first meal was digested.

Drinks after meals (Anupāna): It is common for some persons to ask for a sweet drink after enjoying a meal of sour items and for others to ask for a sour drink after a sweet meal. An appropriately chosen post-prandial drink would facilitate digestion, revive the relish for food and remove fatigue. A physician would choose a drink after meals for a patient based on his disease, time of the year and components of his meal. Among the various drinks, rainwater is the best because it contains all the six rasas.[24]

From a long list of post-prandial drinks recommended, a few representative samples are given in Table 13.[25]

Table 13: Selected Postprandial drinks for different foods

Food	Drink recommended after meal
Cereals	Juice of jujube fruits
Pulses	Sour gruel
Meat of swift runners (jāṅgalyas)	Pippalyāsava
Meat of peckers (viṣkira)	Āsava of kola and badara
Meat of tree dwellers (vileśaya)	Phalāsava
Meat of riverine fish (nādeyamatsya)	Āsava of lotus stalk
Meat of sea fish (sāmudramatsya)	Āsava of mātuluṅga
Sour fruits	Āsava of kamala and utpala
Sweet fruits	Khaṇḍāsava with trikaṭu
Pungent fruits	Āsava of dūrvā, nala and vetra
Greens of pippalyādi group	Āsava of gokṣura and vasuka

In conclusion, water is an appropriate drink after any kind of meal. If the drinks mentioned in the list are taken at the beginning of the meal, it would lead to loss of weight; if taken during the meal, weight would be unaffected; as an after drink, it would enhance body weight. After drinks are not advised for those with diseases of the head and neck, hoarseness of voice, and chest wound.

References:

1. *CS Sūtra* 25: 5 - 40
2. *CS Sūtra* 25: 31
3. *CS Sūtra* 25: 40 – 41
4. *AH Kalpa* 6: 5 -7
5. *AH Sūtra* 7: 1 – 18
6. *CS Sūtra* 27: 3

7. *CS Sūtra* 27: 8 – 22
8. *CS Sūtra* 27: 23 – 34
9. *CS Sūtra* 27: 35 - 60
10. *CS Sūtra* 27: 88 - 124
11. *CS Sūtra* 27: 125 - 165
12. *CS Sūtra* 27: 166 - 177
13. *CS Sūtra* 27: 178 - 195
14. *CS Sūtra* 27: 217 - 236
15. *CS Sūtra* 27: 237 - 249
16. *CS Sūtra* 27: 250 - 285
17. *CS Sūtra* 27: 286 – 308
18. *CS Sūtra* 27: 332 – 341
19. *CS Sūtra* 5: 4
20. *AH Sūtra* 8: 46
21. *CS Sūtra* 27: 350
22. *SS* Sūtra 46: 446 – 448
23. *SS Sūtra* 46: 449 – 457
24. *SS Sūtra* 46: 419 – 422
25. *SS Sūtra* 46: 433

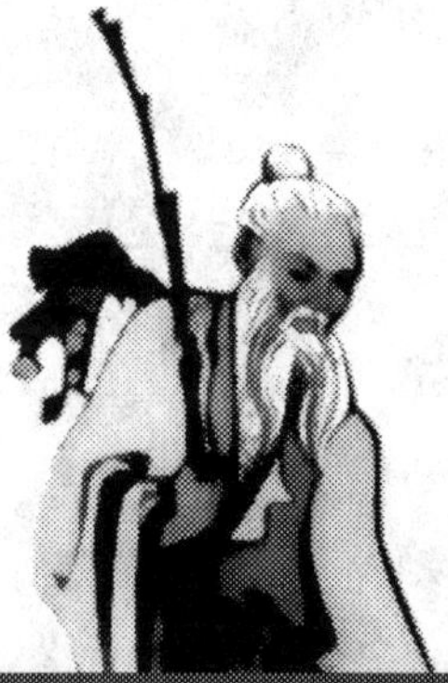

CHAPTER 8

A Code for Living

A code for healthy living is often referred to in Āyurvedic texts. Observance of the code is essential for maintaining good health (svasthavṛtta), for enjoying a full life span without infirmities, for living at peace with oneself and all other living beings, and for ensuring a life of bliss hereafter. The ancient code was widely observed in India, because it appears in varying forms in Bṛhattrayī and resonates even today in popular literature and an average citizen's life in India. It is however, largely applicable to the middle class as many instructions may be beyond the capacity of the poor to comply with. The economic facts of healthcare are ignored in medical texts regardless of whether they were written two thousand years ago, or even today. Alone among ancient authors, Caraka does make a solitary reference, when he recommends an elaborate set of procedures for emesis and purgation for the Kings and rich individuals; but adds, "The poor too in case of a disorder requiring evacuation may take the drug even without collecting the rare equipment. Because all men do not have the requisite means and it is also not that severe diseases do not attack the poor. Hence, one should take, in case of affliction, the treatment and also the clothes and diets according to his means."[1]

The injunctions of the code of conduct cover a wide range of activities extending from the earthly to the spiritual, from the tangible to the intangible and the individual to the universal. The injunctions and directions of the Āyurvedic code will be considered under two broad categories.

Code for mundane living

Good health is the best source of righteous conduct, wealth, fulfilment of desire, and emancipation (puruṣārthas). Diseases rob these attainments from life, if not destroy life itself.[2] To safeguard good health from predators, an individual should always remain vigilant and take a number of measures as outlined below:

Daily Code: One should wakeup three hours before sunrise, which signals the auspicious moment of Brāhmamuhūrta. The waking up should trigger a short introspection when one should ponder on the endless flow of days and nights and how one's existence figures in the course of circadian events. This is the recipe to the cessation of sorrow.[3] After easing oneself and cleansing properly, one should brush the teeth with the crushed tips of the twigs of astringent, bitter, or pungent plants such as arka, nyagrodha, and khadira, taking care not to hurt the gums.[4] Tongue should be scraped regularly with scrapers made of metals.[5]

Eye care should be done daily by applying a collyrium of sauvīrāñjana, which moistens the eyes, sharpens vision, and promotes the growth of eye lashes.[6] A collyrium of rasāñjana is recommended additionally, once a week to promote lachrymation and removal of kapha accumulation. Thereafter, nose drops, medicated smoke, and chewing betel with camphor and cloves should also be done as per textual recommendations. Medicated smoking, herbs used for making the smoking formulation, procedure, benefits, and necessary equipment were described in detail by Caraka.[7] The application of anutaila as nasal drops also received Caraka's endorsement. All these measures were believed to prevent a variety of nasal and upper respiratory disorders. Oil massage of the body and bath should be done every day and the application of oil was especially important on the head, ears, and feet. In these daily practices, care should be taken to spare those who suffer from kapha-induced and other ailments and a physician should be consulted for advice.

Physical activity was encouraged as it has multiple benefits such as improvement of digestion, reduction of adipose tissue, and enhanced stability of the body. The optimum level of physical activity and the dangers of over-exertion were indicated.[8]

Massage has several merits as it reduces kapha, dissolves adiposity, and makes the skin supple. Similarly, regular bath improves appetite and digestive power, and promotes long life and strength. While warm water is good for bathing the body, it may be harmful for washing the head, lest it should hurt the eyes. Bath may not be advisable for patients with various diseases and a physician should be consulted for advice. Sweating is an indication of a satisfactory level of physical activity.

After bath, wearing of comfortable clothes, garlands, and precious stones, and the application of sandal paste on the body were advised. This is auspicious and a source of pleasure and cheer to the individual.[9] Regular haircut and paring of nails thrice in a fortnight, using footwear and carrying umbrella and stick during walks were recommended.[10] After the morning rituals and bath, worship of gods, guests, and Brāhmaṇas was mentioned in a general way but no hymn, rituals, or place of worship were highlighted.

Sleep was discussed in great detail. Sleep during the day and night, the necessity for sleep, the debilitating effect of the lack of sleep, sleep of old people and children, sleep in patients with serious diseases, and other aspects of interest to the physicians were considered elaborately before concluding that "a normal person should sleep regularly at night and if he must keep awake at night, he should sleep for half that period the next morning on an empty stomach."[11]

Sexual intercourse: Vāgbhaṭa's instructions on sexual intercourse were detailed and dealt with the theme in the manner of a clinical manual. It indicated the appropriate timing, locations, frequency, and so on, and included a long list of prohibitions. For example, sexual intercourse was suggested every third day except in summer, when the frequency was reduced to once a fortnight. It was forbidden in women during periods, who lack libido, are filthy, belong to a higher caste, are sick, or are of the same family. Subject to the restrictions, healthy sexual activity enhances memory, intellect, life expectancy, health, strength, repute, and freedom from senility.[12]

Regarding food, one should eat only after the previous meal is digested. The meal should be agreeable and moderate in quantity so that it gets digested in time even if it contains heavy items. The proper quantity would ensure that the consumed food stimulates the digestive fire for both heavy and light items in the diet. Inadequate quantity would deplete strength and cause vātaja disorders; excess would increase the doṣas and cause perturbation.

Attitude to tradition: Tradition as beliefs, opinions, and customs handed down by generations and reaching back to the beginning of civilisation always had a strong hold on the Indian mind. When tradition was reinforced by universal respect for preceptors, the practice of questioning old beliefs and customs became rare. On the other hand, the questioning of authority or established doctrines was always vigorous in India and most outstanding exemplar of this movement was Lord Buddha who repudiated the authority of the Vedas. But the practice of learned criticism did not trickle down from philosophy to traditional events in the common man's life. The Saṃhitas of Caraka and Suśruta have plenty of "dos and don'ts," which would illustrate the kind of daily life that people were enjoined to live.

- One should worship gods, cow, Brahmanas, preceptors, elderly people,[13] and noble teachers; Should offer oblations to the fire, wear auspicious herbs, bathe twice a day, clean excretory orifices, and feet frequently; wear simple and neat clothes, flowers and use perfumes; sport hair style seen in common practice; apply oil to the head, ear, and feet daily; use medicated smoke, open conversations in company, and remain cheerful; maintain equanimity in trying circumstances; pray at road crossings; perform religious sacrifices, offer hospitality to guests and rice balls to one's ancestors; speak meaningful brief, and sweet words; be in control of senses and intent on cause and not the effect; remain free from anxiety, fear, and shyness; be brave, skilful, forgiving, spiritually inclined, and optimistic; be of noble conduct; avoid dirty places littered with garbage, hair, ash, bones, and places of sacrifice and bath; stop exercise before fatigue sets in; be fraternal, tolerant of others' harsh words, and avoid the extremes of attraction and repulsion; prize peacefulness and shun intolerance.

- One should not scale mountains or climb trees or sport in swift currents; not laugh loudly, pass flatus noisily, yawn/sneeze/laugh with open mouth; not pluck the nose, grind teeth, crack fingers, strike bony prominences, scrap the earth or disturb earthen mounds, or assume abnormal postures of the body; should avoid the sight of unholy and inauspicious objects, or wail aloud on seeing a dead body; should not remain in places of worship, raised platforms, cross roads, cremation grounds at night, or enter abandoned houses; not make friends with women, acquaintances and servants with sinful conduct, not be rash, slothful, or gluttonous; not be aggressive to wild animals with conspicuous teeth and horns; not eat without wearing jewels on the hand, before taking bath, with torn clothes, without chanting mantras, and without offerings to gods, ancestors, preceptors, guests, and servants; not eat without washing hand, feet and face and rinsing mouth, facing north, or gloomy in attitude with faithless, dirty and hungry attendants; not eat from unclean plates in awkward and crowded places at improper times; not take preserved food except meat, salad, dry vegetable, fruits, and hard edibles; eat liberally except for curd, honey, salt, roasted grain, flour, and ghee; desist from taking curd at night; not sneeze, eat or sleep in abnormal position; not do extraneous things, or face wind, fire, water, moon, sun, Brahmanas, or preceptor while easing oneself; not urinate on the road; not blow the nose during the chanting of mantras, offering of oblations to the fire, studies, and auspicious acts; not insult women or repose too much faith in them or let them into secrets or invest them with authority; not procrastinate when action is needed but not act without prior thinking; not be a slave to senses or the fleeting mind; not overburden the senses, or act under the stress of anger or jubilation; not be a victim of prolonged grief, or yield to the exhilaration of success, and despair of failure; be confident of the objective of action, which must be initiated without delay; never lose courage.

Seasonal code: Bṛhattrayī texts were composed in north India where the extremes of weather in summer and winter would dictate suitable adjustments in life style. Known as "ṛtucarya," this evolved from a set of lifestyle changes into a doctrine based on the concept of equilibrium between the body and the external environment (ṛtusāmya). A year was divided into six seasons of two months each, and Āyurveda grouped the six seasons into two equal halves. The first half consisting of śiśira, vasanta, and grīṣma was termed as ādāna, when the sun would draw away moisture from earth and all life forms. As water sustains life, ādāna would witness the depletion of body strength of animal and man, withering of plants and the general attenuation of life. As salt water in a bowl exposed to the sun becomes more concentrated, it appeared to the ancient observers that body chemistry would undergo similar changes with a rise in the concentration levels of bitter, astringent, and pungent rasas in the body fluids (rasa was the ancient term for chemicals, hence rasatantra for chemistry). After the desiccation of ādāna, the second half of the year or visarga consisting of varṣa, śarat, and hemanta would follow. During this period, the sun's power would decline, clouds would gather and bring forth rain and return whatever was taken away from earth during ādāna. During visarga, earth would cool, living beings would regain strength, and sour, salty, and sweet tastes would dominate the body fluids (Figure 1). The responses of the body to the changed environment outside would involve doṣas and dhātus, which are constituents of the body. This would manifest in behavioural changes in sleep, appetite, energy level, physical activity, and libido which are well known. A code of conduct to suit the seasons was accordingly prescribed, covering diet, bath, clothes, massage, travel, sexual intercourse, application of cooling paste on the body, enjoyment of wine, and many other activities of daily life. The prescribed diet and life style during each half of the year was based on the principle that seasonal changes would produce alterations in the chemistry of body fluids, which would inevitably be reflected in doṣa perturbation. These were sought to be countered by the prescribed diet and life style. Table 1 explains the rationale for the change of conduct during the two halves of the year (ādāna and visarga).

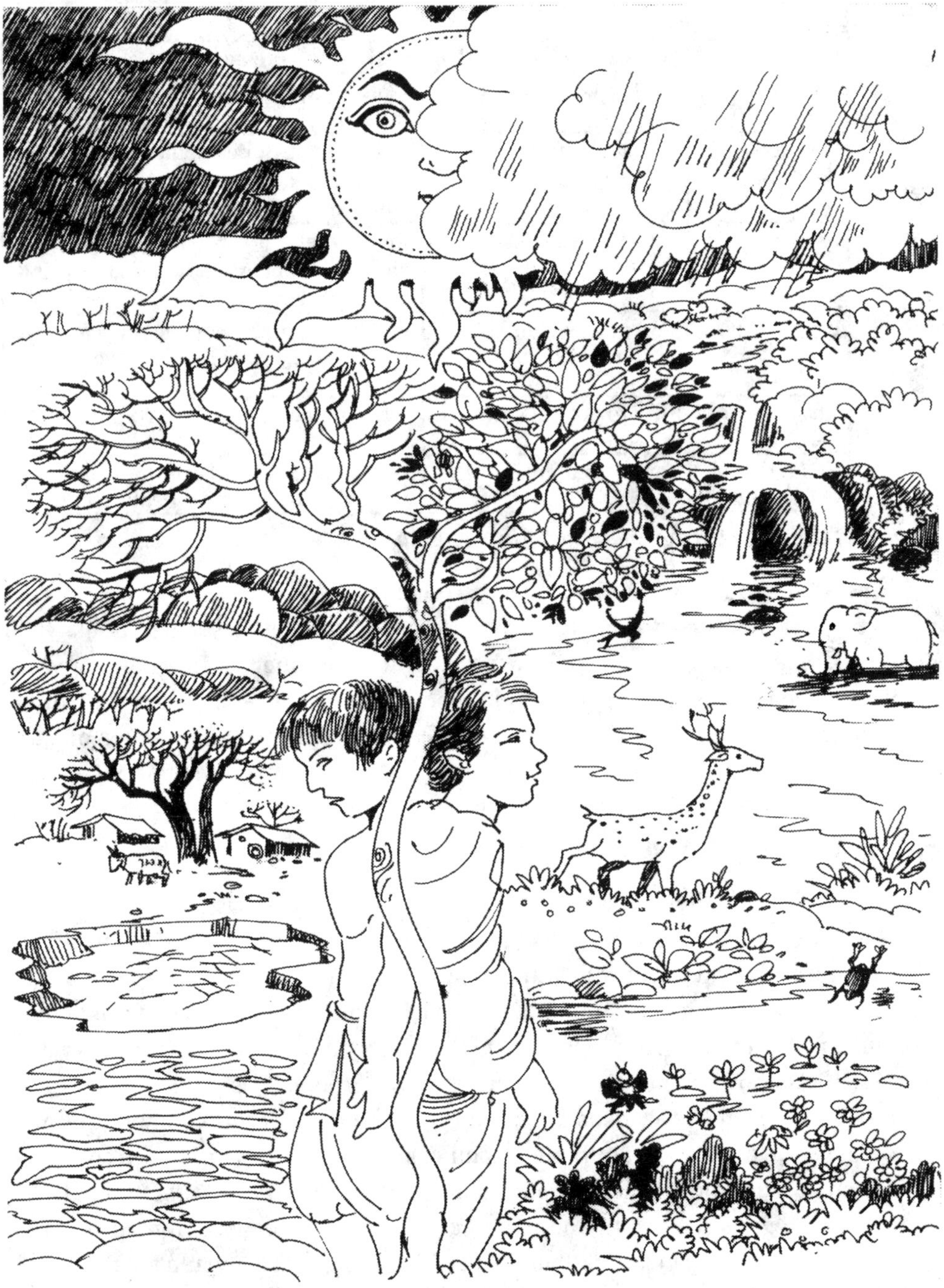

Figure 1: Ādāna and Visarga (Dry and Wet halves of the year)
Ādāna (Left): Moisture drawn away from earth; life withers
Visarga (Right): Moisture returns; life breaks out in celebration

Table 1: Doṣas, Diet and seasonal changes

	Season	Doṣa Status	Diet/other measures
Ādāna	Śiśira (late winter)	Kapha accumulates	Same style of food and activity as for early winter (hemanta)
Ādāna	Vasanta (spring)	Kapha to be evacuated	Spicy, rough, pungent, alkaline, astringent food articles; vigorous exercise
Ādāna	Grīṣma (summer)	Vāta accumulates perturbs	Sour, sweet, salty articles, ghee, milk, sugar; avoid heavy manual activity and wear light clothes
Visarga	Varṣa (rain)	Vāta perturbed to be evacuated; pitta accumulates	Astringent, bitter, pungent articles; sleep in a dry place: avoid travel
Visarga	Śarat (autumn)	Pitta to be evacuated	Astringent sweet, bitter articles; light clothes
Visarga	Hemanta (early winter)	Kapha accumulates	Salty, alkaline, bitter, sour pungent articles; warm clothes; heated room

Details of the table are given in the Suśruta Samhita[14]

It is important to recognise that ṛtucarya recommended for seasonal adjustment in North India is not applicable as such to other parts of India, such as Tamil Nadu or Kerala, where the extremes of weather between summer and winter is absent. A different challenge in ṛtucarya in our time is how to develop a mechanism for maintaining the equilibrium between the body and the surroundings when one can reach Trivandrum from Delhi in four hours in December when the temperature in Trivandrum would be 25°C with humidity of 60 percent and Delhi would be freezing at 10°C with a humidity of 30 percent.

Code for Virtuous living

The code for mundane activities including daily and seasonal codes is specific to location, time and cultural traits of the people. The code for virtuous living, on the other hand, transcends the mundane and reaches out to values which are eternal and universal. Among living beings, it is the singular dignity of humans to value certain ideals above comfort, wealth, health, or even life. This human trait makes Āyurveda a philosophy that goes beyond medical sciences, because it identifies man as not merely a living and admirable machine, but also as the symbol of a collective aspiration of mankind. A perfect policy based solely on a code for mundane living would give humans the health and happiness symbolized by a contented cow in a herd; but this would be incompatible with the life of humans; it would fail to achieve a form that will last for thousands of years. The kind of living that humans aspire for is not limited by the mundane code which guarantees physical vigour, health, and a sense of well-being; instead, it is a condition best suited to reach goals that may bear no relation to biological necessity or usefulness. The prize which humans crave most, and which often inflicts scars of suffering, have determinants which are not mundane and are not completely accounted for by scientific laws. This is exemplified in history by humans who were driven, regardless of consequences, by powerful ideas in arts, religion, and politics. In the Āyurvedic view, alone among living beings, humans are willing to subordinate the purely biological manifestation of existence to a higher form of life conceived in dharma (righteous conduct).[15, 16]

Caraka describes good conduct which he terms "sadvṛtti" and regards it essential for the "maintenance of health and control for senses."[17] Āyurveda proclaims that the overuse, underuse, and misuse of senses is the principal cause of diseases.[18] Caraka's directions on virtuous living are however mixed with instructions on many mundane issues relating to the body and social behaviour of individuals.[19] But his statements are direct and can be outlined as:

- "One should not tell a lie or covet another's property or women; should not harbour enmity against anyone; should desist from sinful acts even against a sinner; should not speak about defects in others or pry into other's private affairs; should shun the company of traitors, lunatics, depraved persons, abortionists and the wicked."
- In the grand oath administered by the preceptor to the trainee physician, Caraka has given the characteristics of a noble physician. The oath gives in great detail a series of injunctions which would bind the student physician in his personal, professional, academic, and social life. In the concluding part, the oath states, "these is no end to Āyurveda, hence one should devote himself to it constantly and without negligence. This is worth doing. Further one should learn without jealousy excellence even from enemies, because for the wise the world is a teacher while for the unwise is an enemy."[20]
- Happiness and misery arise due to contact of the self, sense organs, mind, and sense objects. But when the mind is focused on the self, both cease to exist and a spiritual power appears in the person. This is yoga which signifies a transformation and the end of misery.[21]

Vāgbhaṭa's stress on the supremacy of righteousness was no less than Caraka's. Consider these statements:[22]

- Every activity of living beings springs from the urge towards happiness. But true happiness cannot be had without righteous conduct (dharma). Therefore, one ought to adopt righteousness in conduct and serve the good and friendly with devotion, while keeping away from the wicked.

- One should shun violence, theft, sexual misconduct, calumny, harsh speech, untruth, divisive talk, harmful thoughts, greed, and impiety which are the 10 sinful acts of the body and mind. Every assistance according one's capacity should be rendered to the indigent, to the sick, and to all those assailed by grief. One should regard even worms, ants, and other creatures as no different from oneself. Reverence verging on worship should be offered to gods, cows, savants, vaidyas, the elderly, kings, and guests. Suppliants for help should never be turned away empty-handed, scolded, or humiliated. On the contrary, one should be generous even to a foe who is bent upon doing harm. Prosperity and adversity should not upset one's equilibrium. Envy should be directed towards the resolve and effort which lie behind success and not towards the successful. No effort should be undertaken which is not conducive to the attainment of righteousness.

- The world is a teacher for a wise individual in all activities and he should keenly observe whatever happens in nature and adapt his action accordingly. Good conduct is no more than having a heart full of compassion, of giving away gifts to the deserving, of possessing control over one's body, speech and mind; and of identifying others' hardships as one's own. The wise man never grieves, who constantly introspects on all his deeds as the cycle of days and nights revolves unceasingly.

Sadvṛtti is the signature tune with resonates through the Āyurvedic panorama.

References

1. *CS Sūtra* 15: 19 – 21
2. *CS* **Sūtra**1: 15
3. *AH Sūtra* 2: 47
4. *AH Sūtra* 1: 4
5. *CS Sūtra* 5: 71 – 75
6. *AH Sūtra* 2: 5 – 8
7. *CS Sūtra* 5: 20 – 55
8. *AH Sūtra* 2: 11 – 15
9. *CS Sūtra* 5: 95 – 97
10. *CS Sūtra* 8: 18
11. *AH Sūtra* 7: 56 – 65
12. *AH Sūtra* 7: 74 – 77
13. *CS Sūtra* 8: 18 – 21

14. *SS Sūtra* 6: 10 – 12
15. *AH Sūtra*2: 20
16. *CS Sūtra* 30: 24
17. *CS Sūtra* 8: 18 – 19
18. *AH Sūtra* 1: 19
19. *CS Sūtra* 8: 18 – 19
20. *CS Vimāna* 8: 14
21. *CS Śārīra* 1: 138 – 139
22. M S Valiathan. *The Legacy of Vāgbhaṭa*. Orient Blackswan, Chennai 2009. Chapter 2: Page 11 – 12.

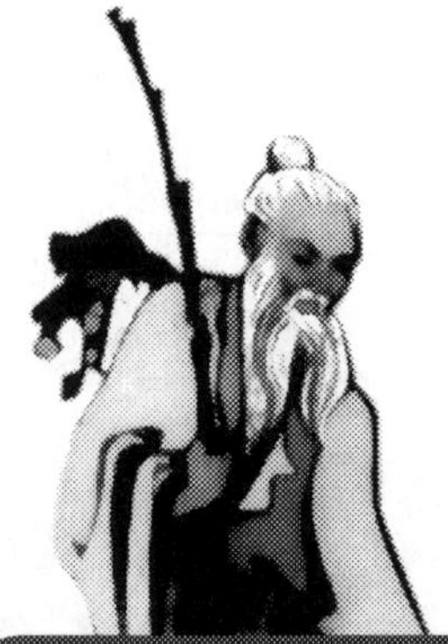

CHAPTER 9

Clinical Medicine

Importance of diagnosis

Many dreaded diseases caused by bacteria, viruses, and parasites have been eliminated in the last hundred years; many others in the non-communicable list are under control and the patients live useful lives for many years. These advances were made possible by the spectacular progress in science and technology and the improved standard of living, thanks to socio-economic progress. Medical students see patients with smallpox and plague no longer, and few with leprosy; patients with fearful diseases of the past such as typhoid fever and pneumonia are safely treated as outpatients or undergo a short hospitalization. In spite of all these and many more advances, hospitals are always full not only in India, but in developed countries as well. The old problems have yielded place to new, which are equally fearsome such as drug resistant TB, AIDS, dementias, mental illness, and many degenerative diseases. As long as this trend continues, the process of making a diagnosis will continue to face every physician as the indispensable first step in treating a patient. In the history of medicine and its practice throughout the second millennium right up to mid-19th century in Europe and India, there were remarkably few tools to analyse or "image" the changes taking place within the body during illness. The dismal picture began to change toward the end of the 19th century when Roentgen discovered x-rays for imaging the body, chemistry made advances to detect the biochemical correlates of diseases in body fluids, and physicists and physiologists took the lead in designing and making electrophysiological instruments. When we look back to the period from first to sixth centuries associated with CS, SS, and AH, one cannot but be humbled by the enormous intellectual effort made by the ancient physicians to make a diagnosis in the absence of tools. Their success was acclaimed by Professor Kutumbaiah, a former Professor of Medicine in the Christian Medical College, Vellore and a pioneer in Ayurvedic studies, who commented on Caraka's exposition on diagnosis "it is perhaps the most comprehensive and complete discussion of the subject of diagnosis we possess in any ancient medical literature including corpus Hippocraticum."

Diagnosis according to Caraka

Diagnosis is held as supremely important in Bṛhattrayī as the three authorities of Āyurveda were united in giving priority for diagnosis in the practice of medicine. Their aim was not to give a label to a disease based on various findings, but to identify a particular state of disequilibrium of doṣas in a patient, which may or may not be known as a particular disease. Vāgbhaṭa says, "a physician should never feel ashamed of being unable to name a disease; the fact is that all diseases have not been named."[1] In this chapter, the discussion on the diagnostic process will be based on Caraka's exposition.

Diagnosis depends on what is observable in the patient by the physician. The disease of the patient may be caused by the inappropriate contact between the senses and their objects, erroneous judgment leading to imprudent conduct (prajñāparādha), or the effect of the passage of time on life.[2] These three causes lead to diseases of somatic origin. They are paittika (pittaja), saumya (kaphaja), and vātika (vātaja). There are two other types which belong to the psychic domain, rājasa and tāmasa. The diagnosis begins with a preliminary assessment of patients.

Preliminary assessment

While treating a patient, a physician may be asked, "How many types of examination do you want to conduct before opting to do pañcakarma or other procedures on this patient? What all examinations would you conduct? How would you conduct them? What is the purpose of your examination? What is to be done and not to be done? To answer such questions, a physician should be fully informed about 10 items relating to the patient, his disease, and treatment. These are discussed below:[3,4]

Kāraṇa (Doer): In the medical context, the doer is a physician and what follows is a list of 10 items related to him and the medical context. The physician is one who triumphs over diseases, who knows Ayurvedic texts and how to apply their maxims. He should ask himself: "Am I competent to re-establish the equilibrium of dhātus in this patient? Do I have the knowledge of theory, practical knowledge, and manual skill (jiṭahastatā)? Do I have all the necessary equipment (upakaraṇa)? Do I possess the ability to control my sense organs and the working of nature?" This exercise in introspection is the key to the physician for treating the patient himself or referring the patient to another physician or specialist for better care.

Karaṇa (Instrument): It means instrument; but in this context, it signifies a drug which, for a physician, is an instrument for re-establishing the equilibrium of dhātus.

However, medical treatment is of two kinds, spiritual and rational (daivavyapāśraya and yuktivyapāśraya). The spiritual employs incantation, roots, gems, fasting, worship in temples, oblations, donations, and so on. The rational has two types; evacuative and pacificatory (saṃśodhana and upaśāmana). The rational can also be viewed as employing material things or psychological means. For example, material things are primarily drugs such as emetics and purgatives; psychological means include frightening, springing surprise, chiding, binding, inducing sleep, and such measures known collectively as "upāyas". These are mostly employed in treating psychiatric patients. Physicians were expected to have or arrange for the supply of appropriate drugs.

Kāryayoni (Source): The source is disequilibrium of dhātus followed by the imbalance of doṣas which occurs in terms of their deficit or excess. This has significance for the curability, curability with difficulty, and incurability of the illness.

Kārya (Purpose): The restoration of the equilibrium of dhātus is detected by the recovery of normal voice, complexion, increase in strength, improved appetite, good digestion, proper sleep, absence of disturbing dreams, effortless awakening, easy evacuation of bowels and urine, and alertness of the mind and intellect.

Kāryaphala (Result): Is happiness arising from recovery which results from the satisfaction shared by mind, intellect, sense organs, and the body.

Table 1: Preliminary Assessment

Kāraṇa	Prakṛti
Karaṇa	Vikṛti
Kāryayoni	Sāra
Kārya	Samhanana
Kāryaphala	Pramāṇa
Anubandha	Sātmya
Deśa →	Sattva
Kala	Āhāraśakti
Prāvṛti	Vyāyāmaśakti
Upāya	Age

Anubandha (Sequel): Longevity after recovery characterized by the union of the body with vital breath (prāṇa).

Deśa (Place): This term is used in two different senses in the diagnostic process. In the first place it means the patient, wherein the disease resides. Secondly, it is also the place where the patient resides. Both these are important for making a diagnosis. This dual meaning of "deśa" will be considered at the conclusion of the present discussion of the 10 items in the preliminary assessment of patients.

Kāla: Time is measured in years and also in the condition of the patient. It can be divided into two, three, six, twelve, or even more parts based on the therapeutic action under consideration. Here, the discussions will be based on division into six months. Hemanta (early winter), grīṣma (summer), and varṣa (rain) have three intercalary seasons which share common features such as prāvṛti (early rains), śarad (autumn), and vasanta (spring). These intercalary seasons are best suited to carry out evacuative therapy.[5]

Prāvṛti: Indicates the initiation of therapy. This is made possible by readying the medical quartet consisting of the physician, patient, medicament, and attendant with the prescribed qualities for each.

Upāya: This refers to the overall excellence produced by the high quality of the medical quartet and the equally high quality of their performance which takes into account all the 10 points mentioned under preliminary assessment and 10 points figuring under deśa. The entire object of this detailed examination is "pratipatti" which is the determination of the specific treatment for a particular disorder.[6]

Discussion on Deśa[7]

Deśa as land: It is important to enquire and know about the land where the patient was born and where he lives, where he grew up and where he became ill, what sort of diet, conduct, strength, mentality, illness, agreeability, and disagreeability do the people have in that location, and what sort of medicinal plants grow in that place. These enquiries would give the physician a good understanding of the patient and his/her geographical, familial, and social background.

Deśa as body: Patient's body is the seat of activity (kāryadeśa). The examination in this category should focus on the possible life span as can be determined by an assessment of the patient's strength and nature of illness. This is essential because the dose and potency of the medicine to the administered should be appropriate to the strength of the patient. If too strong dose of a potent medicine is given to a weak patient, that would be harmful. The potent medicine in this context includes oral medications and also procedures such as cauterization and surgical procedures. While a highly potent medicine may hurt or even kill a weak patient, a medicine of low potency or doze may be ineffectual in a strong patient. Therefore, the patient's strength should be carefully assessed in terms of prakṛti (constitution), vikṛti (disturbance in equilibrium), sāra (the status of dhātus), saṃhanana (compactness of dhātus), pramāṇa (body measurements), sātmya (compatibility), sattva (mentality), āhāraśakti (digestive power), vyāyāma śakti (exertional power), and age. These are discussed below:[8]

Prakṛti: The prakṛti of an individual is determined at the time of conception in utero. The doṣas – one or more – are attached to the foetus at the moment of conception. This is what gives an individual a characteristic constitution or doṣa prakṛti. The prakṛti may be vātala, pittala, or śleṣmala. They have characteristic features which are briefly outlined below:

- *Vātala:* Associated properties are: rough, light, mobile, plentiful, fast, cold; coarse; short and thin body; rough skin and hoarse voice, poor sleep; unsteady movement; variable diet, speech and activities; talkative; quickly irritable, fearful, equally quick in attachment and aversion; quick in acquisition and loss of memory; intolerance to cold; coarse hair, skin, nails, teeth, face, hands, and feet; clicking joints; low in strength and wealth, few progeny, and low in life span.
- *Pittala:* Intolerant to heat; delicate body and body parts; hot face; moles, discoloured patches, pimples on the skin; severe hunger and thirst; early wrinkles and greying of hair; soft, few and brown beard and short hair; intense, sharp, stray; enjoys plentiful food and drinks and frequent eating; highly mobile joints and muscles; much perspiration, urine, and sweat; fleshy smell and odour in axilla, mouth, and body; moderate in strength, knowledge, wealth, and life span.
- *Śleṣmala:* Individuals with śleṣmala or kapha prakṛti have organs which are smooth and well lubricated; body and organs soft, delicate, and felicitous; abundant semen, fecundity, and sexual prowess; organs well developed, solid and compact; indolent, slow in activities such as eating, and speech; slow in initiating activities or getting irritated; poor appetite, hunger, and perspiration; strong joints and ligaments; clear complexion and amiable voice; strong, learned, wealthy, fearless, and long life span.

  A patient should be examined, keeping in mind the characteristics of the three prakṛtis, which may be mixed in different individuals with dominance of one or the other.

Vikṛti: This is a manifestation of disordered prakṛti. It should be examined from the standpoint of the strength of the cause, perturbed doṣa, dhātus involved, place and time, which are manifested by symptoms. When the characteristics of disease and of the perturbed dhātus are synergistic, the disease manifestation will be severe; if not, it will be mild.

Sāra: Sāra is the essence of tissues, including dhātus, which is the source of their strength. It is determined by the presence of characteristic signs in the body which a physician can detect. The tissues are skin, blood, muscle, adipose tissue, bone, marrow, semen, and mind. For example, the signs of the sāra of skin are smoothness, softness, clarity, lustre, and warmth; sparse, deep-rooted, and delicate hair; the sāra of skin suggests happiness, good fortune, power, enjoyment, intelligence, learning, health, jubilation, and long life. Physicians may mistake a subject to be strong by finding him of large size and weak because of his small size, which may be false in both cases. This kind of mistake could be avoided by careful attention to the examination of sāras of tissues on the basis of their manifestations.

Saṃhanana (compactness): This is a state when the various parts of the body are joined together tightly and harmoniously to serve body functions. The parts include bones, joints, muscles, and blood. Compactness makes an individual strong; its absence makes one weak; those with moderate compactness have medium strength.

Pramāṇa (measurement of body parts): The persons with normal measurements of body parts have long life, strength, resistance to diseases, happiness, dominance, prosperity, and other merits. The values of the measurements of the whole body in terms of height, breadth, and length are stated in detail and the measure used is "finger breadth." This is a standard source of reference for Ayurvedic physicians.[9]

Sātmya (compatibility): It is a quality, which enables an individual to attain well-being by finding compatibility with food (e.g.: milk, ghee, oil, meat, soup etc.) and with all the six rasas. Sātmya confers strength and long life. Those who find compatibility with a single rasa and coarse food items will be low in strength and short in life span.

Sattva: Signifies the mind which, in union with self, regulates all body functions. Its strength is rated as high, medium, or low. The high type has memory, devotion, gratitude, limpid eyes, courage, skill, fighting spirit, resolve, sharp intellect, and virtuous conduct. Though they may be of short stature, they maintain equanimity in internal or external crisis; those with medium strength survive on the support of others; and the low cannot survive either on their own or with the support of others. They are unable to bear pain or suffering in spite of possessing a big body.

Āhāraśakti: It indicates one's ability to eat and digest food. This is the basis for sustaining the body.

Vyāyāmaśakti: It indicates one's capacity to undertake physical activity or work.

Age: Counts the changing status of body over time. It has three periods – childhood, middle age, and old age. Childhood counts up to 16 years when dhātus are immature, sexual functions are latent, body parts are soft, strength is underdeveloped and kapha is dominant. This stage may continue up to 30 years with an immature mind. Middle age is shown by strength, virility, power, procurement and retention, eloquence, qualities of dhātus in full display, mental strength, and dominance of pitta. This lasts up to 60 years. Next comes old age up to 100 years when dhātus, virility, power, procurement and retention, memory, speech, and comprehension decline and vāyu gains dominance. These characteristics ranging from prakṛti to age counterpoised against the three degrees of perturbed doṣas in diseases would enable the physician to determine the strength of medicaments as strong, medium, or low.

This brings us to a close of the discussion on deśa and takes us back to the next stage of diagnosis after preliminary assessment.

Clinical assessment

The preliminary assessment of the patient including the examination of "deśa" are specific to Āyurveda, but the next part of the patient's examination has much in common with the clinical diagnosis in modern medicine. Clinical assessment involves the interrogation of the patient on his complaints, symptoms and their duration, previous history, family history and personal habits, which are followed by physical examination. This involves all the senses of the physician, except taste, which is tested indirectly. Caraka recalls his views on the means to access knowledge, which had been discussed in the chapter on philosophical ideas and applies them in the context of clinical assessment.[10] The physician would gain much knowledge about the patient and his illness by perception of what he sees, hears, smells and feels, which alone may give a tentative diagnosis. For example; pallor is seen, wheezing respiration is heard, gangrene is seen and smelt, and fever is noted on feeling the patient's skin (Table 2). If the patient's urinal attracts a horde of ants, it is a fair guess that he has sweet urine (madhumeha).

Table 2: Diagnosis

Physical examination included the use of all senses: examples	
Eye	Seeing colour, deformities, facial appearance, and size
Nose	Smell of suppuration, sores; cadaveric smell
Ear	Bowel sounds; abnormal breath sounds; crepitus
Skin	Warmth/coldness, colour, goose pimples
Taste	Not directly tested

Next to perception, inference plays a significant role in diagnosis. To employ inference, however, one must have observed the event earlier. The clinical methods of inference – past from the present, present from the past and one from a complementary pair are frequently used by physicians. Examples are sexual intercourse from pregnancy and heavy smoking from coronary artery disease. In addition to perception and inference, Āyurveda laid emphasis on the counsel of saintly physicians who were regarded as "āptas" of profound knowledge, long experience in the practice of medicine and invincible integrity. Their views had as much validity as those from the physician's examination. In some respects, their counsel had a unique benefit for the patient, because it would save the physician from repeating mistakes, which might have been committed by an earlier generation of physicians. Caraka gave an independent role to yukti (reason) as a means to accessing knowledge.

Staging of disease in diagnosis: The diagnostic exercise in Āyurveda paid special attention to the incipient stage to the full-blown presentation of the disease in a patient. They recognized early stages in the evolution of the disease when medical intervention would be more effective. The six stages in the evolution of a disease described by Suśruta had been discussed in chapter 6.

Clinical diagnosis - social aspect: In the India of Bṛhattrayī, people lived in villages separated often by distances or forested land. If a patient fell ill and a physician lived nearby, it was quite common for a relative or a friend of the family to approach the physician on behalf of the patient. These messengers (dūtas) had to be chosen carefully, as a messenger who was intellectually or morally deficient was regarded by the physician as an inauspicious start of a consultation. Though messengers conveyed the report of illness, it would appear that the physician would make a domiciliary visit to the patients' residence and examine the patient before prescribing therapy. The domiciliary visits, the omens connected with the physician's journey and entry into the patients' home were described by Caraka.[11] Diagnosis was made during the visit and it is a reasonable guess that the patient would be transferred to a house for treatment[12] in case he needed pañcakarma or other major procedures.

The diagnostic process was obviously thorough and called for considerable intellectual effort and long clinical experience. These two requirements for diagnosis have not changed notwithstanding the passage of centuries and advances in medical science.

Prognosis

This was of great importance to the physicians as the patient and his family would be concerned and frequently anxious about the question: "what would happen to me from this illness?" Caraka exhorted physicians to assess whether the patient's illness was curable, curable with difficulty, or incurable during the preliminary examination itself. The assessment influenced his therapeutic strategy. To make the assessment, he had to consider the gravity of illness in terms of the perturbation of one or more doṣas, patient's physical and mental strength, and season. He also had to form an idea of the patient's life span from observations. On this point, Caraka and Suśruta were agreed. Many observations were made by Caraka (Table 3), who divided them into those relating to the individual directly and those which did not.

It is significant that while the observations in the left column refer to sense organs, cleanliness, conduct, facial expression, food habits etc., of the patient which could have a bearing on life span, the observations in the right column are not directly related to the patient and are, excepting outcome, based on popular beliefs. It is equally significant that Caraka while urging physicians to examine the patient for items in the left column using perception, inference, and savant's counsel just as he would do for making a clinical diagnosis, also cautions them to interpret the observations in the right column based on authoritative teachings and one's own discretion.[13] He recommended physicians who had observed signs of impending death not to disclose the news without having been requested for. Even when asked for, he should refrain from disclosure if it is likely to precipitate the patient's death or adverse events.[14]

Table 3: Things to be looked at to determine the remaining Life Span

Things relating to the individual	Things not relating to the individual
• Sense organs and their objects • Cleanliness • Conduct • Facial expression • Intelligence • Food habits • Digestive capacity • Physical activity • Dreams	• Messenger approaching the physician • Reflection • Bad omens on the way of the messenger as well as physician • Strange circumstances in patient's residence • Outcome of treatment

References:

1. *AH Sūtra*12: 64
2. *CS Nidāna* 1: 3– 4
3. *CS Vimāna* 8: 85 – 92

4. *CS Vimāna* 8: 125 – 130
5. *CS Vimāna* 8: 126
6. *CS Vimāna* 8: 132
7. *CS Vimāna* 8: 92 – 124
8. *CS Vimāna* 8: 94 – 123
9. *CS Vimāna* 8: 117
10. *CS Vimāna* 4: 3 – 8
11. *CS Indriya* 12: 9 - 24
12. *CS Sūtra* 15: 6 – 9
13. *CS Indriya* 1: 4
14. *CS Indriya* 12: 62 - 64

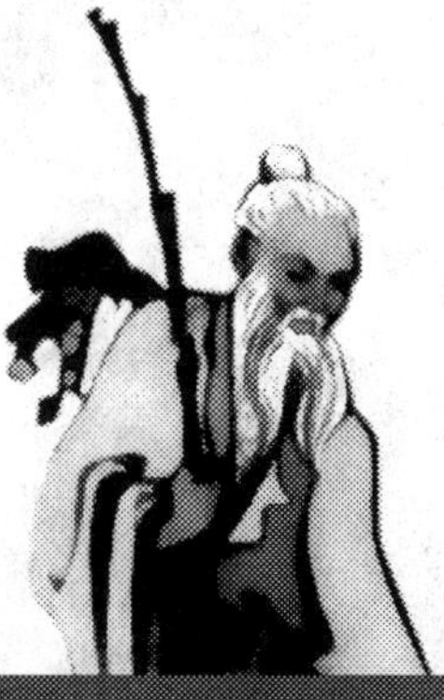

CHAPTER 10

Medical Treatment of Diseases

As soon as the diagnosis is made, the step which follows is the planning and implementation of treatment. Unless there are clear reasons for surgery, patients are always managed by medical treatment, which is the first option. This principle was well accepted by Caraka, who recommended referral of patients to the surgeons – Dhanvantari School as he called them – only when necessary. The need for such referral was obvious in cases of trauma, conditions affecting the eye, women for delivery, and gynaecologic conditions. Specialities existed in Āyurveda which had specialized texts for eye disease, paediatrics, obstetrics, and poisoning.

Medical Quartet: For the optimal treatment of a patient according to Āyurveda, it is mandatory to have a medical quartet in place.[1] The quartet consists of a physician, drugs, attendant, and the patient, each member of the quartet possessed of prescribed qualities. The physician should have sound theoretical knowledge, manual skill, and cleanliness; drugs which include items in the patient's dietary regimen should be available in plenty and should be efficacious, resistant to pests and noxious agents, and amenable to being made into appropriate formulations; the assistant should know how to prepare the drugs and dietary items, how to nurse the patient with skill and compassion, how to maintain hygiene and remain loyal; the patient on his part should remember the details of the onset of his illness and should have candour towards the physician, fearlessness, and readiness to comply with the physician's instructions. Among the quartet, physician will be the leader just as a powerful nation with army and weapons cannot win a battle without an able general. Each member of the quartet was required to have the four essential qualities and given the total of the 16 qualities, the quartet was bound to succeed in their medical mission.

Caraka laid special emphasis on the physician and his responsibility in undertaking to treat patients. A physician who recognizes a disease only partly would be ineffective in treating the patient at best or would be dangerous at worst. If he misjudges a mild illness for a serious disorder and prescribes strong medications and vigorous evacuative therapy, the patient's condition would deteriorate; conversely, if he mistakes a serious ailment for a mild disorder, his therapy would do harm to the patient.[2] As the leader of a team, a good physician should not only possess masterly knowledge and skill, but also possess friendship and compassion towards the ill, joy in treating those whose illness is curable or curable with difficulty and resignation towards those whose disease is incurable. These are indeed the four yogic vṛttis or qualities acclaimed as maitrī, karuṇa, mudita, and upekṣā (friendship, compassion, joy, and resignation).[3]

A house for therapy:[4]

Caraka described a residential facility for patients who needed in-house procedures such as pañcakarma and special kinds of body fomentation. The house was designed and built by architects with special knowledge of vāstu. Safe from strong wind in a valley or flat land, the building would be strong and well ventilated with water reservoir, kitchen, bathrooms, and lavatory. It would have ample room to move about without being harried by sun, rain, dust, and smoke. It would provide accommodation for the patient, physician, and assistant with provision for store and performance of procedures. It would also provide rooms for the stay of musicians and balladeers, whose music and stories would brighten the atmosphere and provide cheer and hope for the patients. The surroundings would be home to birds, roaming cattle, and water bodies. Caraka recognized that treatment of a disease was not merely a therapy for the disease, but also the treating of the whole person.

Curability as a factor in patient selection: During the preliminary assessment of a patient, the physician was obliged to make a determination on whether the disease was curable, curable with difficulty, or incurable. While every effort would be made to save the patient "as long as life breath remained in the throat," Caraka favoured resignation toward the incurable patient who was beyond hope. He was against the prolongation of death in moribund patients with resulting anxiety and agony to the family and attendants. The decision on curability and incurability was made on certain criteria which are indicated in Table 1.[5] It may be noticed that the criteria took into account not only the physical condition of the patient, but also the season, which could be the biting cold or boiling heat of North India.

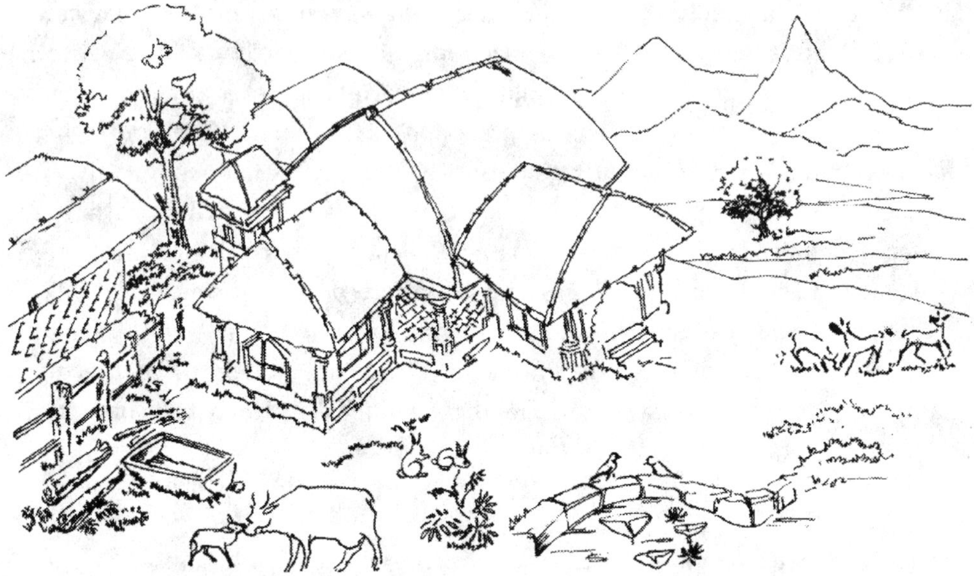

Figure 1: House for Treatment: The design of the building is based on the pattern of residences in 1st century CE in the Kuṣāna Empire; based on photographs of carvings in Mathura Museum (American Institute of Indian Studies, Gurgaon).

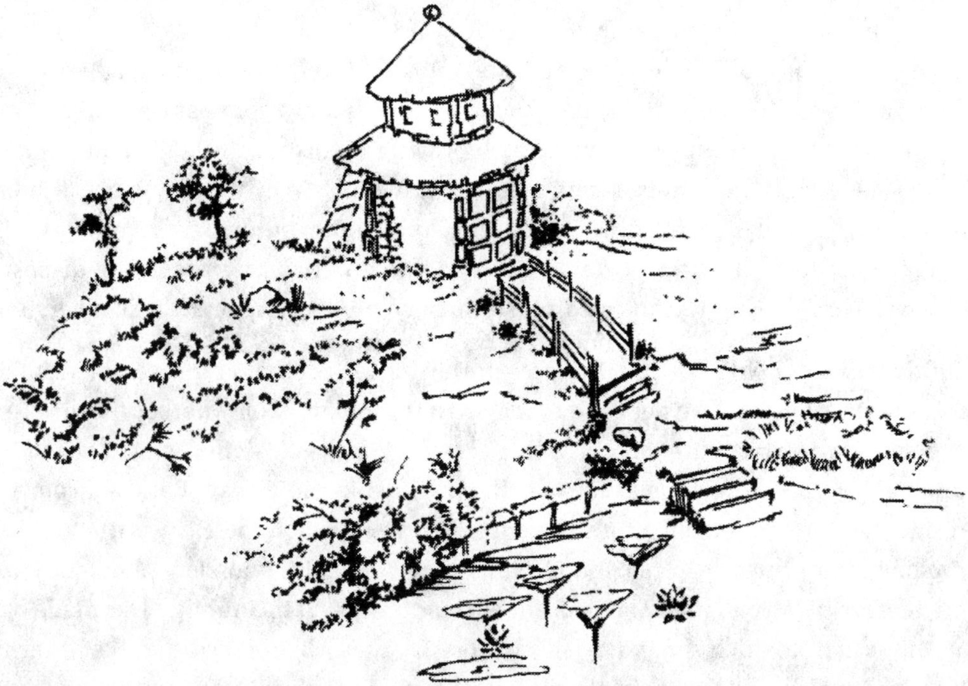

Figure 2: Jentaka (Chamber fomentation): Note the raised location on the bank of a lake and the central chimney; patient was placed in the circular space around the chimney.

Table 1: Curability and Incurability

The issue was decided on the basis of various criteria. They are listed as follows:	
Category	**Criteria**
Curable	Cause, clinical features mild; disturbance of doṣas not amenable to aggravation by the patient's constitution or by season; treatment not impeded by location of patient; only one part affected; disease early with no violent symptoms; one doṣa mainly disturbed; medical quartet in place
Curable with difficulty	Cause/causes, prodroma, symptoms, medium; season, nature of body constituents and derangement of doṣas not synergistic; subject elderly, a woman or infant; symptoms not severe; surgery not necessary; course chronic; affects a vital part, a major joint or only one or two parts; medical quartet not complete; disease not very old; two doṣas deranged
Incurable	Disease lodged in marrow and other deep tissues; many parts including vital organs and joints affected; two or three doṣas deranged; patient debilitated, stuporous; beyond hope of surgery

Guiding principle of medical treatment: During one of the many interesting seminars reported in CS,[6] Maitreya asked Ācarya Ātreya critical questions with reference to the medical quartet. "In spite of the quartet being complete, patients do die; in the absence of all the 16 qualities of the quartet, patients do survive; these are common observations. Therefore, therapeutic measures may have, in fact, no value." To this provocative question, Ātreya gave a detailed answer, in the course of, which he enunciated the principles of treatment as follows:[7] "We treat a sick patient with sickness-relieving therapy; the wasted with wasteness-relieving therapy; we saturate the emaciated and the weak; we treat the obese with reducing therapy; heat with cold therapy and the cold with hot therapy; we restore the depleted dhātus and reduce the amassed dhātus. Thus, by addressing the disorders with techniques opposed to the causative factors, we reestablish the sāmya state." This principle of treatment, it may be recalled, harks back to the vaiśeṣika categories of sāmānya and viśeṣa, which Caraka had modified to indicate that substances with common properties agglomerate, whereas those with opposing properties tend to reduce.

Choice of therapeutic regimen: This is another important principle relating to the choice of a therapeutic regimen which applies to all patients regardless of the causation or location of the disease. The choice of the regimen depends on the severity of illness.

One of the classifications of diseases is based on their severity, which divides them into mild and severe. This simple classification underlies the everyday practice of Āyurveda. In mild disorders, which do not involve major perturbation of doṣas and its manifestations, the treatment is known as śamana. If the perturbation of doṣas is severe and the patient is ill, the elimination of the perturbed and accumulated doṣas will be necessary by a procedure named śodhana.

Śamana: In Āyurveda, health is a state of equilibrium (sāmya) and an important component of it is the equilibrium of agni which is active in all the seven dhātus and most importantly, in the stomach. Agni is constantly "burning" a variety of substrates including doṣas and any slow-down in agni would lead to the accumulation of doṣas in the channels (srotas) which permeate the entire body. Activating the agni (dīpana) is the primary objective of śamana. This is achieved by fasting which, by depriving the fuel of food to agni and lightening the load on agni, enables it to digest the accumulation of doṣas in mild disorders. This practice was known even to common people in India as the Chinese pilgrim Hiuen Tsang reported many centuries ago. Fasting alone may bring relief to the patient, characterized by the return of appetite, feeling of lightness of the body, and belching being free from odour and bad taste. The role of fasting in enhancing the digestive power of agni was recognised in ancient India, and it underlies the practice of various customary fasts. In this kind of fast, the subject is permitted to take only water, coconut water, and clear drinks. An old saying claims that fasting uses hunger as a weapon to treat minor disorders!

Other measures employed in the śamana method are light physical activity, which stimulates agni and enjoying mild sunshine and breeze. These simple activities should be accompanied by agreeable company, rest, and reassurance. There are several other measures such as oil massage, fomentation, and others, which are used in different regions of the country as part of śamana.

Śodhana: The physician should review the status of the patient in a week and decide whether to continue, or modify the treatment, or opt for śodhana therapy to eliminate the excess doṣas which are perturbed and which obstruct the channels in the body (srotas). As the perturbed doṣas contain waste products, which could be toxic, their elimination is regarded as a detoxifying procedure. Pañcakarma consists of five procedures, which are lubricant therapy, fomentation, emesis, purgation, and enema. In head and neck diseases, nasal purgation will replace purgation. Initially the physician would administer an oily formulation chosen based on the patient's strength, bowel habits, and symptoms. The administration of an oily preparation, diet, and management of the patient during lubricant therapy and fomentation, and the complementary procedures of pañcakarma should be done under the supervision of an Ayurvedic physician as complications may occur under unsupervised therapy.[8]

Lubricant therapy is followed by body fomentation in pañcakarma. By fomentation, "Vāta is won over and thus faeces, urine, and semen are never obstructed."[9] It also liquefies the perturbed doṣas in body channels which are loosened following lubricant therapy. Fomentation aids the drainage of liquefied doṣas into the gut as body channels dilate under the effect of moist heat. Three days after lubricant therapy and following body fomentation, the patient should be given a properly chosen purgative by the physician.[10] The choice of patients based on indications and contra indications, complications and their management, and other details of pañcakarma are described by Bṛhattrayī with slight variations. If the patient's disorder is located above the diaphragm, the evacuative procedure following lubricant therapy and fomentation is emesis, if below the diaphragm, purgation or enema, and in the head and neck, nasal purgation. The foregoing account of pañcakarma is presented through a series of box presentations below:

Pañcakarma as detoxification therapy:

- When vāta, pitta, and kapha are perturbed and in excess, they become toxic and call out for elimination. This involves five procedures (pañcakarma) which may be chosen and carried out by a competent physician.
- The five procedures are:
  - Lubrication (Snehana)⁺;
  - Fomentation (Svedana)⁺;
  - Emesis (Vamana);
- Purgation (Virecana);
  - Nasal purging (Nasya);
  - Enema (Vasti) - (Two types: Snehavasti and Kaṣāyavasti)
- Though bloodletting is included in pañcakarma, it is not often used and is excluded by Caraka. This is logical because pañcakarma seeks to eliminate toxic doṣas, whereas bloodletting eliminates a body component (blood), which is vitiated by doṣas.

⁺Essential preparatory steps for all pañcakarma

Preparatory Steps:

Lubrication (Snehana):

- Lubrication or lubricant therapy does not refer to the external application of oily substances; it refers only to internal administration in pañcakarma.
- Lubricants may be of vegetable (sesame, castor) or animal (ghee) origin. Ghee is the best in so far as it settles vāta and pitta, cools, and softens the body.

- The lubricants are mixed in small dozes with other substances; when tolerated well, they may be given alone in larger dozes.
- They loosen and mobilise doṣas which tend to clog body channels.

Fomentation:

- Follows lubricant therapy before pañcakarma is done.
- Excludes local fomentation; whole body fomentation using one of the 13 methods is employed.
- Fomentation is also used independently for treating a variety of diseases including asthma, catarrh, wry neck, hoarseness of voice, and phthisis.

Evacuative Procedures:

Emesis:

- Lubricant therapy and body fomentation must precede.
- Have a bath, wear good clothes, sport ornaments, offer prayers, and be cheerful.
- Comfortably seated, when emetic is taken.
- A friend or attendant should be in attendance.
- Sweating indicates liquefaction of clogged doṣas; goose-flesh indicates their mobilisation and migration from body compartment to the gut (koṣṭha).
- When nausea appears, he should be verbally and physically induced to vomit.
- Signs of satisfactory emesis and post emetic regime indicated.

Purgation:

- Similar to emesis in preparatory steps.
- Purgative drug chosen by the physician to address the patient's disorder, doṣa, prakṛti, season, etc.
- Signs of satisfactory purgation, post-purgation management not very different from those of emesis.
- Caraka, alone among ancient authorities, recommended a "no frills" version of pañcakarma for the common man.

Nasal purging:

- Recommended for diseases of head because nose is the door way to the interior of the head.
- Preparatory steps of lubricant therapy and fomentation identical.

- Performed once, twice, or thrice a day; or following other evacuative procedures.
- Procedure involved applying medicinal preparation through the nose, retention for short periods as prescribed and elimination through the mouth.
- Prompt improvement in many symptoms of head and neck diseases.

Enemas:

- Of all forms of medical therapy, enemas are the most effective; far better than purgation.
- Enemas used not only for evacuation, but also for drug administration.
- Two types – lubricant (snehavasti) and non-lubricant (kaṣāya vasti). The former is secondary and the latter primary.
- Common medium for enema fluid includes devadāru, elā, kuṣṭha, etc.; specific drugs for diseases of patients added when necessary for specific effects.
- Detailed description of enema apparatus, procedure, indications, fluid composition, etc.
- Vaginal and urethral irrigation included under the rubric of enemas.

Mechanism of action of Pañcakarma

Several procedures in Āyurveda such as pañcakarma and rasāyana impress an observer by the imaginative hypothesis which underlies them. They are not products of empiricism where a procedure which originated in the distant past and found to work reasonably well is followed faithfully by the succeeding generations as a part of traditional medicine. Hypothesis involves an exercise in creative imagination to find an answer to a problem on the basis of observed facts which are by themselves a puzzle. A gifted individual contemplating an observation, turning over various images and ideas in his mind on what was observed would come upon a novel scheme which would seem to solve the puzzle in hand. The next step for a scientist would be to test the scheme in a scientific experiment, whereas a physician would test the novel idea in patients in ancient times. In the case of pañcakarma, the perturbed doṣas clogging the body channels, lubricant therapy loosening them, hot fomentation driving them into the gut - none of these were observable; they were products of the creative imagination of India's ancient physicians. When they tested the imaginative scheme in patients, it worked and became an established procedure, which continues to be in vogue thousands of years later. No wonder, Vāgbhaṭa says confidently, "this science of Vedic origin (Āyurveda) has demonstrable results and is fit to be used as a mantra with no room whatever for doubt."[11]

Treatment of Mental Illness

Mental illness was recognised as a branch of medicine and called bhūtavidyā, which figures in the Chāndogya Upaniṣad. Caraka believed that mind had its own channels in the body (manovāhika srotas), which were connected with the dhamanis arising from the heart. According to Āyurveda, heart is the seat of consciousness, emotions, and all cognitive functions. If the mental channels of the heart get clogged with perturbed doṣas that would start a process which would lead to insanity.

Mental illness was divided into five types – one each dominated by vāta, pitta and kapha and the fourth by three doṣas together. The fifth type was caused by totally external causes.[12] In weak-minded people, many undesirable activities such as: eating unclean food, practice of tantric rites, adopting body contortions, and yielding to excess of anger, greed, jubilation, anxiety, fear, and grief hurt the mind, and perturb doṣas, which block the mental channels to the heart and cause mental illness. Mental illness (unmāda) is defined as involuntary roaming of the mind, intellect, consciousness, knowledge, memory, conduct, and activities. Its prodromal symptoms include emptiness of head, excited eyes, ringing in the ears, rapid breathing, salivation, aversion to food, tightness in the chest, meditation, fatigue, goose flesh, puffiness of face, and several behavioural traits which look abnormal.

Onset of the disease is marked by frenetic movement, frequent movements of eye brows, and arms, unceasing and incoherent talk, salivation, irrational jubilation by singing and dancing, and other activities. In vātaja insanity, irritability and anger, irrational excitement, inflicting injury on oneself and others with weapons, desire for coolness and shade, congested eyes, dislike of heat, and other symptoms are seen; in pittaja type, preference for solitude, silence, inactivity, drooling of saliva, and nasal discharge; and liking for sleep, puffiness of face, and moist and dirty eyes are the features of kaphaja type of insanity. In the sannipāta type, clinical features from the three types are mixed.[13]

The exogenous type of illness is quite different from the types caused by doṣa perturbation. This type may be the effect of karma or the acts of imprudent conduct due to the error of understanding (prajñāparādha). These acts of misconduct or erroneous conduct include insult to gods, teachers and forefathers, which invite effects in the form of insanity with varied manifestations. A feature of this type of insanity is extraordinary power, courage, bravery, overpowering intellect, and eloquence and unpredictable explosions of insanity. It is believed that unholy and profane acts which cause this type of insanity occur at certain times of vulnerability and under certain circumstances. These are described in detail.[14]

It is noteworthy that following a long discussion on the type of insanity caused by offended gods and supernatural agents and the punishment decreed by them in the form of serious mental illness, Caraka adopts a different, if not defiant, attitude when he states;[15] "No gods, gandharvas, piśācas, or rākṣasas nor others would torment an individual, unless he or she has made oneself vulnerable by their own misdeeds (prajñāparādha). One should desist from blaming gods, forefathers, and others when a disease strikes because of one's own erroneous understanding and conduct. One should regard oneself as the creator of one's own happiness and unhappiness."

Treatment of mental illness:[16] In brief, the types of insanity caused by perturbed doṣas are treated by therapeutic measures similar to the treatment of somatic disorders caused by the perturbation of doṣas. For example, in vātaja variety, mild evacuative procedures following lubricant therapy; in the pittaja and kaphaja varieties, emesis, and purgation are administered following lubricant therapy and fomentation.

There are also dietary regimens and many formulations recommended for patients following their evacuative measures. In managing patients with doṣa-induced diseases of the pittaja and vātika types, the physician may be faced with violent and uncontrollable patients. Under such circumstances, he should not hesitate to prescribe extreme measures such as frightening, beating, touching with bristles of kapikaccu and massaging with mustard oil and binding.[17] He could also be terrorized by exposing to edentulous snakes, trained lions, or elephants, which are innocuous. These frightful methods have no place in treating insanity caused by insolence towards gods, teachers, and forefathers. Such patients should be treated by milder medications and by inducement to worship, making donations, chanting of hymns, conducting rituals of expiation, and other sacred acts.[18] Above all, sincere and daily worship of Lord Siva, the master of Bhūta attendants and Lord of the earth would overcome insanity.

References

1. *CS Sūtra* 9: 3 - 12
2. *CS Vimāna* 7: 4 – 7
3. *CS Sūtra* 9: 26
4. *CS Sūtra* 15: 5 - 7
5. *CS Sūtra* 10: 7 – 20
6. *CS Sūtra* 10: 4 – 5
7. *CS Sūtra* 10: 6

8. *CS Sūtra* 13: 62 – 64
9. *CS Sūtra* 14: 3 – 5
10. *CS Sūtra* 13: 80
11. *AH Uttara* 40: 81
12. *CS Nidāna* 8: 3 – 45
13. *CS Nidāna* 7: 61 – 63
14. *CS Nidāna* 7: 10 – 14
15. *CS Nidāna* 7: 19 – 23
16. *CS Cikitsā* 9: 24 – 32
17. *CS Cikitsā* 10: 79 – 84
18. *CS Cikitsā* 10: 87 – 91

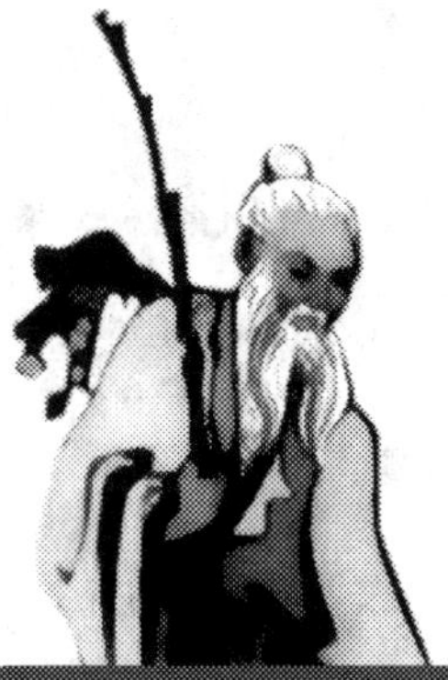

CHAPTER 11

Drugs (Dravyas) and Taste (Rasa)

"Dravya" - a drug - has three types; a pacifier of doṣas, a vitiator of dhātus, and a promoter of healthy living.[1] Āyurveda employs drugs as medicinal preparations extensively in many forms and Caraka Saṃhitā (CS) classifies them in the very first chapter into those of vegetable, animal, and earthy origin. The entire chapter is devoted to a detailed description of 600 evacuative drugs and their characterization. Western physicians and rulers such as Garcia da Orta and Van Rheed, and scientists such as Roxburg and Ainslie, who took interest in India's traditional medicine laid primary emphasis on medicinal plants. The studies in Āyurveda by modern science from 16th to the better part of the 20th century CE were dominated by taxonomy, pharmacology, and natural products chemistry of medicinal plants. The fascination continues undiminished even today in India and abroad, and there are entire institutes and university departments dedicated to research in medicinal plants. CS is believed to have mentioned 1900 medicinal plants, of which less than 1000 have been identified unanimously (Ved). Similarly, over 1000 herbal formulations are in the market and are expanding in number.

To survey the vast field of drugs in Āyurveda within the confines of this chapter it is necessary to formulate a plan and stick to essentials. The plan is as follows:

- Classification of drugs;
- Drug action and taste;
- Basics of drug action; and
- Ayurvedic Pharmacy.

Classification of drugs[2]

Substances of vegetable, animal, and mineral origin dominated medical therapy in India, China, Egypt, and Greece. In India, Vedic medicine relied mainly on medicinal plants in the treatment of diseases. Numerous hymns in the Atharvaveda were addressed to medicinal plants for the recovery of patients as their beneficent effect was believed to take place through supernatural forces. As Indian plants such as cinnamon, pepper, and ginger are mentioned in corpus Hippocraticum, the basis of Greek medicine composed in 500 BCE, a trade existed between India and Greece in the ancient world. The plants were used in Greek medicine and praised for their good effects. In India's ancient Gurukulas where young physicians received training, they acquired thorough familiarity with plants including their identification, regional variations, cultivation, preservation, methods for making formulations, and toxic manifestations. After six or seven years of training in a Gurukula, they would enter practice on their own with a mastery over the subject of medicinal plants.

Drugs of vegetable origin: These drugs belong to four types viz: vanaspati, known by fruits; vānaspatya, by flowers and fruits; oṣadhi, by the plants dying after fruiting and vīrudh, by growth by spreading. Six trees are included in this list, snuhi, arka, aśmantaka, pūtika, kṛṣṇagandha, and tilvaka though they differ from the plants because of their special usefulness in evacuative therapy. The parts of plants used for therapy include bark, root, heartwood, secretions, stalk, juice, tender leaves, latex, fruit, flower, ash, oil, thorn, leaves, leaf buds, tubers, and sprouts. Caraka lists 16 plants with useful roots and 19 with useful fruits, which were probably the most commonly used drugs for evacuative purposes. This is a small fraction of the total number of plants mentioned in CS, which rated medicinal plants growing in Himalayan Valleys as the best and most efficacious.

Drugs of animal origin: In terms of thc variety and frequency of use, animal products follow at a great distance after medicinal plants. Examples are honey, milk and milk products, bile and bile stones, muscle, fat, marrow, blood, faeces, urine, skin, semen, bone, ligament, horn, nail, hoof, and hair. There is however little doubt that items like ghee, milk and milk products, and honey dominate animal products in Āyurveda.

Drugs of earthy origin: Examples are gold, pañcaloha (silver, copper, iron, lead and tin), silica, calcites, realgar, orpiment, gems, salts, ochre and galena (note the absence of mercury). Drugs of earthy origin constitute the smallest part of Ayurvedic formulary. Whether mercury in Āyurvedic rasaśāstra was indigenous in origin or imported from West Asia is controversial.

The relative prevalence of these three varieties of drugs in different parts of the world was greatly influenced by geographical factors. Thanks to arid conditions, West Asia used minerals and metal derived products widely, whereas plant derived drugs held sway in India.

Drug Action - Taste

Rasa (taste) is a central concept in Āyurveda. It should at once be distinguished from "rasa" derived from ahārarasa, which conveys nutrients to the dhātus in the body. Taste signified chemistry in ancient India and "rasa" was used, more or less, as a synonym for chemistry. When chemistry made its advent in India centuries later, it was appropriately named "rasatantra"! The importance of taste for the practice of medicine was such that a vigorous discussion on rasa is reported in detail in CS, where the topic received critical attention.[3] The discussion opened with Bhadrakāpīya postulating one rasa only to Kankāyana insisting that rasas are innumerable! Ācārya Punarvasu intervened at this stage and declared that there are six rasas, which are: sweet (madhura), sour (sour), salty (lavaṇa), pungent (kaṭu), bitter (tikta), and astringent (kaṣāya). These rasas reside in substances (dravyas) composed of five bhūtas, which remain constant though the rasas may be mixed in the substance (Table 1).

Consisting of five bhūtas, drugs may be sentient or non-sentient and their properties include 20 ranging from heavy/light. Their actions are five evacuative functions such as emesis. The actions of drugs which are derived from five bhūtas reflect the properties of the parent bhūtas (Table 1).

Table 1: Therapeutic effect of drug substances

Drugs	**Bhūta-based properties**
Purgatives	Earthy, watery; moves downward
Emetics	Fiery and airy: moves upwards
Pacifying drugs (Śamana)	Ethereal
Digestive	Fiery
Lightening	Airy and fiery
Building	Earthy and watery

A glance at Table 1 shows that earthy, watery purgatives move downwards; fiery, airy emetics move upwards, etc. It is on this ground that a statement is made that there is no substance in the universe which cannot be used as a drug provided it is used rationally.[4]

However, the action of a drug is not limited to its bhūta lineage or its taste experienced in the mouth. The action may be influenced by the varying changes of the dravya with time, the locations where the changes take place and the purpose for which the changes are brought about.[5] What the changes do is action (karma), the means by which they act is potency (vīrya), where they act is the place of action (adhikaraṇa), when they act is time (kāla) and how they act is mechanism (upāya) and what they achieve is result (phala). When this sequence is translated into the course of a drug following its intake by mouth, we would find a corresponding sequence of events on the following lines. A physician administers a drug possessing one of the six primary tastes as dominant and some others as secondary tastes which are 63 in number. He may administer substances with tastes singly or in combination to suit the clinical condition of the patient.

As the drug gets digested in the stomach, it undergoes changes and the means by which these changes are brought about is potency (vīrya). These changes are physicochemical because the digestion in the stomach makes the drug mucoid and frothy, but at the same time, its taste would also change from its primary taste at the time of ingestion. One gets an indication of this chemical transformation of a substance in the stomach from the change in the taste sensed during belching. This transformation would continue as the assimilable part of digested drug moves further in the gut and ultimately reaches the dhātus. The taste – "the final taste" of Suśruta or vipāka – is attained when the assimilable part reaches the dhātus to provide replenishment.

Post-digestive Taste (Vipāka):

- ✓ During digestion in the stomach by the action of "jaṭharāgni", dravya undergoes physical changes such as liquefaction, mucinous appearance etc.; it also undergoes chemical changes, which are shown by the change in taste (rasa) of the material. The taste of an item in the mouth and during belching illustrates this. The post-digestive taste when the assimilable part of ingested dravya reaches dhātus is vipāka.
- ✓ Rasa indicates taste; vīrya represents potency which transforms ingested substances; vipāka represents the final taste when action impinges on dhātus.

The vipāka, "final taste" of Suśruta, is a far cry from the primary taste from which it evolves. In other words, the choice of drugs with properties opposed to those of the perturbed doṣas is not simple like the administration an alkali to counter an acidic substance because of the series of changes, which a substance undergoes from the time of ingestion to the point when the assimilable part of drugs possessed of vipāka reaches the dhātus. The dhātus are the ultimate place of action (adhikaraṇa) as the desired result of the entire exercise is to carry the essence of the drug to the dhātus and cause addition or diminution according to the law of sāmānya and viśeṣa. The effect of drugs with their inherent tastes and dominant bhūtas on the doṣas is shown in Table 2.

Table 2: Effect of drugs on doṣas (with inherent tastes and bhūta dominance)

Taste (Inherent in drugs)	Bhūta Dominance	Effect on Doṣas	Bhūta Dominance	Taste (inherent in drugs)
Sweet, Sour, Salty	Earthy, Fiery, Watery	Pacify → Vāta ← Perturb	Airy, Fiery, Ethereal, Earthy	Acid, Bitter, Astringent
Sweet, Bitter, Astringent	Earthy, Watery, Airy	Pacify → Pitta ← Perturb	Earthy, Fiery, Watery, Airy	Sour, Salty, Pungent
Pungent, Bitter, Astringent	Ethereal, Fiery, Airy	Pacify → Kapha ← Perturb	Earthy, Watery, Fiery	Sweet, Sour, Salty

Lastly, it must be noted that substances may act on patients in ways which cannot be explained on the basis of taste, potency, and post-digestive taste or vipāka alone. A good example given by Vāgbhaṭa is dantī which is no different from citraka in taste, but dantī is a purgative which citraka is not. There are many other examples including the wearing of charms.[6]

Inexplicable action (Prabhāva):

- ✓ It is observed sometimes that the effect of a particular substance on a patient cannot be explained on the basis of taste, potency and post-digestive taste. The effect may even be dramatic. This is termed "prabhāva," which is a special effective action.
- ✓ Prabhāva would explain phenomena such as a substance with a characteristic taste produces a certain effect, while another with a similar taste fails to produce the same effect. It would also explain how the sporting of precious stones produces beneficial effects in certain individuals.
- ✓ In a trial of strength, post-digestive taste (vipāka) overcomes rasa, potency subdues both, and prabhāva triumphs over all three.

Basics of Drug Action

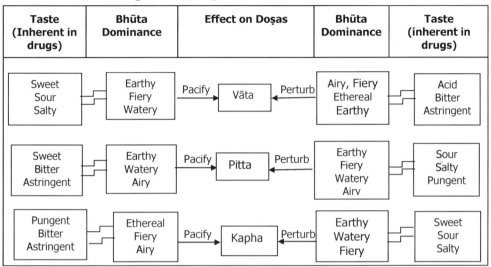

Therapeutic action of dravya or drug was of great interest to ancient physicians in India. Plants which produce diverse actions such as emesis, purgation, and sedation grew in the same locale, shared the same climate and yet produced very different responses in the human body. As noted earlier, Caraka adopted 20 qualities (guṇas) from vaiśeṣika system for dravyas (substances) which comprehended drugs. The qualities used by Caraka[7] were heavy/light, cold/hot, moist/dry, smooth/rough, slow/fast, solid/liquid, soft/hard, immobile/mobile, subtle/gross, clear/turbid, which were of obvious importance in the making and use of drugs. These qualities were inherent in substances by the law of samavāya[8] and once they are taken away, the substances would lose their identity. There was a great deal of discussion and even disagreement among Ācāryas on the question whether the therapeutic effect of a particular dravya was due to the dravya per se or to the quality (guṇa) inherent therein.[9] The controversy does not seem to have over-riding importance today for physicians who may take the view that the substance and the particular quality under review are after all inseparable.

However, the ancient debate was as much philosophical as medical and was summed up by Suśruta as follows: "The dravyas, their tastes, potencies, and final tastes indicate their individual importance as upheld by their supporters. The learned, however, regard all these four views (substance, taste, potency, and final taste) as equally important. Some drugs vitiate or eliminate doṣas by their own actions, some by their potencies, and some by their tastes and final tastes."[10] Suśruta concluded, "as the final taste (vipāka) is not possible without potency (vīrya) which brings about actions such as emesis and purgation, potency is not possible without taste (rasa), and taste is not possible without drug (dravya), drug should be regarded as supreme."[11]

Effect of Drugs on doṣas

Vāgbhaṭa said, "Vāta, pitta, and kapha are the three doṣas; in equilibrium, they sustain the body and in disequilibrium, destroy it."[12] A physician called upon to treat a patient with a disease and attendant disequilibrium of doṣas must know the drugs which would counter the disequilibrium. Table 2 indicates, tastes grouped on the basis of their inherence in drugs and their bhūta dominance with their effect on the three doṣas. If a patient is found by the physician to have a vāta or, pitta or, kapha induced disorder, he would be obliged to choose a drug on the basis of its taste and bhūta dominance. The information in Table 2 is a key to make this determination, which would however have to be fine-tuned by other factors.

There are other factors which influence drug action. An example is time reflected in season when the patient ingests the drug, in the stage of the patients' disease, and in the age of the patient.[13] Each one of these manifestations of time would influence the action of drugs on the patient.

Ayurvedic Pharmacy

As mentioned earlier, over a thousand herbal drugs are believed to be sold in the Indian market and the number is steadily rising. As each herbal drug contains several, if not many, medicinal plants it is obvious that many hundreds of plants are currently being used in the treatment of patients. Though taken for granted, this is a most remarkable achievement. To be included in the Ayurvedic formulary, a plant has to be identified from nature's stupendous garden of hundreds of thousands of plants, perhaps ten percent. Barring regional practices in India, it is doubtful whether any plant not mentioned by Bṛhattrayī has been added to the Ayurvedic formulary by their successors in the next 15 centuries. Once a plant is identified, its activity has to be located in some or all of its parts; a process has to be developed to convert it into a polyherbal formulation, taking care to enhance their pharmacologic synergies and neutralize toxicities of components; a suitable method of storage – safe from pests and extremes of seasons – has to be invented; it will have to be cast as pills, licks, and so on to suit the heterogeneous likes and tastes of patients. The gigantic effort involved in developing the present Ayurvedic formulary documented in over 50 authoritative texts is a truly herculean achievement.

The following outline on the making of herbal drugs in ancient India is based on descriptions of Vāgbhaṭa and Sāraṇgadhara.

Harvesting herbs:

Some of the ideal conditions and locale for the collection of herbs are: arid country in temperate zone, smooth land, and fertile soil; far away from cremation grounds, monasteries, highways, having lakes and water bodies not far away, where kuśa and rohiṣa grow in plenty, uncultivated land and with no big trees. The plants should have grown in natural surroundings and have healthy colour, should grow vigorously with roots pointing to the north.[14]

The person to collect plants should be clean in mind and body and should fast the previous evening. If the plants from the ideal locale and conditions are not available, herbs not more than a year old should be collected with a few exceptions like sugarcane, pippalī, and viḍaṅga.

Caraka's directions are similar, but he classifies the locale as dry, marshy, and intermediate in terms of merits for the collection herbs.[15] In this connection, Caraka's caution to physicians on the understanding of herbs is apposite. He states "It is not, however, by knowing plants by names and forms that one understands medicinal plants fully. He would have full understanding, who knows not only their names and forms, but also knows how to administer them according to the place and time and the individual constitution of the patient."[16]

We have seen the standard classification of drugs based on origin – plant, animal, and minerals. Sāraṇgadhara who lived in the 14th century gave a different and lucid classification of drugs based on their pharmacological action. Examples are given below:[17]

Table 3: Classification of drugs-Pharmacological Action

Classification of drugs	*Comment*
Dīpana (appetizers) E.g.: Mishi	Stimulates digestive fire in stomach; does not cook food
Pācana (digestives) E.g.: Nāgakeśara	Cooks undigested food
Anulomana (aperients) E.g.: Harītaki	Expels flatus and faeces after full digestion
Sraṃsana (laxatives) E.g.: Kṛtamalaka	Expels flatus and faeces–digested and undigested
Bhedana (purgatives) E.g.: Kaṭuki	Breaks up faecal mass and expels with flatus
Vamana (emetics) E.g.: Madanaphala	Expels raw pitta and kapha from stomach through mouth

The list includes over 20 pharmacologic actions including madakāri of alcohol and vyavāyi (quick general diffusion) of bhang. The principles of the administration of the drugs are also specified.

Drug preparations:

The drug is prepared in different forms to suit the patient who may be a child, adult, edentulous, apprehensive, weak, and so on. Sāraṇgadhara lists 12 preparations as follows:[18]

Table 4: Drug preparations and its descriptions

Drug preparations	**Descriptions**
Svarasaadhyāya	Fresh juice
Kvāthakalpana	Decoctions
Phaṇṭakalpana	Infusions
Himakalpana	Cold Infusions
Kalka kalpana	Wet pills
Chūrna kalpana	Powders
Guṭika kalpana	Pills
Avalehakalpana	Confections
Snehakalpana	Medicated oil/ghee
Sandhānakalpana	Galenicals
Dhātuśodhana - māraṇakalpana	Purification and preparation of minerals and metals
Rasādi Shodhana - māraṇakalpana	Mercurials

Each of the above groups is dealt with in a separate chapter in a business-like manner for practicing physicians. Drugs were largely administered orally: but rectal (enema), nasal (nasya), and transdermal (medicated oils) routes were also used frequently.

Sāraṇgadhara Saṃhitā also gives details on the measures employed in making formulations, methods of preparation and duration of potency of drugs on storage. It concurs with Vāgbhaṭa that drugs from Himalayan country are "saumya" and those from Vindhya are "agneya."

Then and Now:

The preparation of drugs in ancient India was often done in the physician's home or Gurukula or in the house of affluent patients. Indigent patients were often supplied medicines free by the physician as compassion was a fundamental requirement for the practice of Āyurveda. However, the stagnation and decline in Āyurveda for centuries prior to and during the British rule in India bore witness to the collapse of many traditions in the training of physicians, service to patients especially surgery, and the development and practice of pharmacy. It is to the credit of pioneers such as Vaidyaratnam P S Varier in Kottakkal, Gananath Sen in Kolkata, and Lakṣmīpati in Chennai that major reforms were adopted against stiff opposition in the training of Ayurvedic physicians through colleges of Āyurveda and the manufacture of Ayurvedic drugs by modern technology in full compliance with the ancient protocol. If the production of herbal drugs claims over Rs 6, 000 crores a year today, government and industry are determined to double or triple that figure soon, and patients can easily obtain the drugs, we have to thank the pioneers who foresaw the need to combine tradition with modernity in the right measure a 100 years ago.

References:

1. *CS Sūtra* 1: 67 - 68
2. *CS Sūtra* 1: 67 – 119
3. *CS Sūtra* 26: 8 - 11
4. *CS Sūtra* 26: 12
5. *CS Sūtra* 26: 13
6. *AH Sūtra* 9: 26
7. *CS Sūtra* 1: 49
8. *CS Sūtra* 1: 50
9. *SS Sūtra* 40: 3 – 4
10. *SS Sūtra* 40: 13 – 14
11. *SS Sūtra* 40: 15

12. *AH Sūtra* 1: 6
13. *SS Sūtra* 41: 5
14. *AH Kalpa* 6: 1 – 4
15. *CS Kalpa* 1: 7 – 9
16. *CS Sūtra* 1: 120 – 123
17. *Sāraṇgadhara Saṃhitā* 1: 4: 1 – 8
18. *Sāraṇgadhara Saṃhitā* 2: 1 - 12

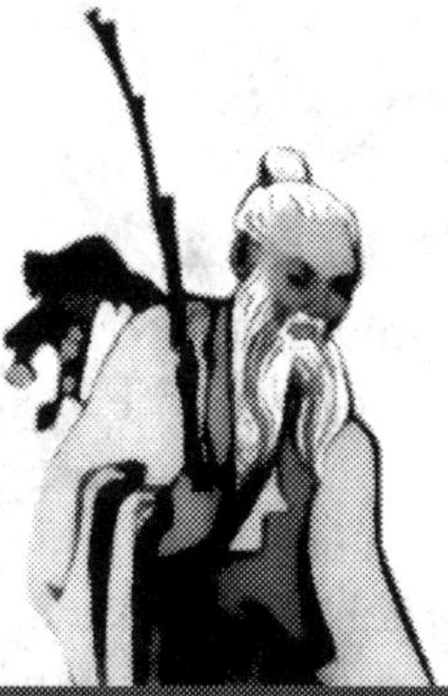

CHAPTER 12

Surgical Treatment of Diseases

Surgery: The first branch of Āyurveda

Surgery is a chapter written in gold in the history of ancient India. It represented the peak of manual skill, medical knowledge, and spirit of daring, all driven by compassion toward fellow beings. Suśruta Saṃhitā opens with a scene, where eager students of Āyurveda including Suśruta were seated at the feet of Kaśirāja Divodasa who was not only esteemed as the King of Kaśi, but also revered as a divine physician and an incarnation of Lord Dhanvantari. The students' sincerity to learn Āyurveda impressed the Ācārya who asked them, which branch of the vast subject they had wished to learn. On being told unanimously that they had chosen surgery (śalya), Divodasa was immensely pleased and affirmed "among the eight branches of Āyurveda, śalya is the best and the oldest, and is attested by the modes of perception, inference, analogy, and scriptural authority. It is the oldest because śalya healed the wound caused by weapons and ferocious animals in times of yore (Figure 1).

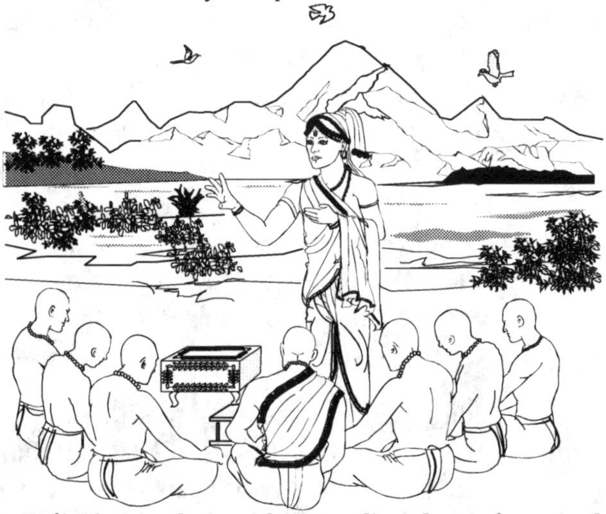

Figure 1: Kāśirāja Divodāsa with seven disciples, Suśruta in the middle

Legend has it that an incensed Rudra severed the head of yajña and, on gods' entreaty, Aśvins reattached the head and were assured in return a portion of the sacrificial offerings by Indra. Śalya is also the most important among the branches of Āyurveda because it produces quick results from the use of instruments, alkali, and cautery, and comprehends all that the other branches contain. It unbars the gates of heaven and is eternal, virtuous, worthy of high repute, and generous in providing a means of living. I am no other than Dhanvantari who saved the gods from decay and death and am born on earth to impart śalya with its allied branches of knowledge to humanity."[1] After this luminous testimony from Kaśirāja-Divodasa, no more need be said about the glory of surgery.

India's surgical heritage is inextricably linked to Suśruta who lived in Varanasi. There is unanimity among scholars that the Saṃhitā which currently bears his name is a redaction of the original by Nāgārjuna in the fourth century CE. Though Suśruta's period is controversial, there is enough reason to believe that he lived prior to the Buddha and blazed a trail in surgery, which had few equals in the ancient world. What follows is a narrative based on the theory and practice of surgery as one finds in Suśruta Saṃhitā.

Surgery in Suśruta's period: As we read the account of surgical operations, treatment of fractures and dislocations, and the conduct of complex deliveries in women, we must remind ourselves of the serious limitations under which surgeons had to function in those far-off days. In the first place, there was no anesthesia anywhere in the world until nitrous oxide was introduced as "laughing gas" by Humphry Davy in England as late as the 19th century. The patient was sedated by heavy doses of wine and was physically restrained by muscular attendants during surgical procedures. As the time available was always short, surgeons had to be quite sure of regional anatomy and highly skillful in the use of their hands. This necessarily restricted the scope of surgery. Secondly, anatomical knowledge was imperfect, because the method of dissection in a rotting cadaver to learn anatomy could never provide exact information of various parts and viscera of the body, which the surgeon needed. The general practice of cremation of bodies could also have discouraged the dissection of cadavers. Thirdly, serious procedures in surgery or treatment of very sick patients carried considerable risk of punishment by the State as indicated by the following:

> Physicians undertaking medical treatment without intimating to the authorities the dangerous nature of the disease shall, if the patient dies, be punished with the first amercement.* If the death of a patient under treatment is due to carelessness in the treatment, the physician shall be punished

with the middle most amercement. Growth of disease due to negligence or indifference of physicians shall be regarded as assault or violence.[2]

* (Fine or any major punishment)

The boundary conditions which governed a surgeon's professional work were so highly restrictive that the surgical achievements of Suśruta become all the more admirable.

Surgical Operations - Pre- and post-operative care: A surgical procedure is an episode in a sequence starting with pre-operative care (pūrva karma), and ending with post-operative care (paścātkarma). This will be illustrated by a commonly done operation of incision and drainage of an abscess.

Pre-operative management:[3] The surgeon should ensure that the array of 100 blunt and 20 sharp instruments, caustic alkali, cautery, surgical horn, and a set of accessory instruments such as cotton, cloth, bandage, bamboo, fan, honey, ghee, medicinal decoctions, ointment, pastes, and plentiful supplies of hot and cold water are arranged and kept in order for use. The operating room, large and well ventilated, should be fumigated prior to the operation. Strong, fearless, and friendly attendants should be available throughout the procedure.

Incision and drainage:[4] The procedure should be fixed on an auspicious day and the patient must fast the previous night. Brāhmaṇas and physicians should be honoured with gifts and hymns chanted prior to the procedure. Patient should face east and should be physically restrained by a strong attendant. The physician facing west, should make an incision quickly in the direction of hairs on the skin, sparing vital spots and major vessels. The incision should be deepened until pus emerges. For this to succeed, the abscess should be mature, fluctuant, and located in an accessible part. Physicians should be clear headed, bold, quick with the use of hands, and free from tremor and sweating. The knife must be sharp. If the incision does not let out pus, careful inspection must be made and an additional incision made to drain it. If necessary, incision should be oblique, arcuate, or near-circular to suit special or awkward locations on the face, axilla, gums, groin, anus, and penis. Mistakes in making incision may result in serious injuries to vessels or other structures and result in delayed healing.

Following the procedure, cold water should be sprinkled on the face and the patient reassured. The wound should be gently massaged to express pus and washed with a medical decoction. A cotton wick soaked in a paste of sesamum, honey, and other drugs should be gently inserted to keep the wound open to facilitate drainage. A medicated paste should be applied over the wick and the wound was bandaged. The bandaged site should be exposed to fumigation which has analgesic and protective properties. A paste made from guggulu, aguru, sarjarasa, vacā, gaurasarṣapa, nimbapatra, salt, and ghee is recommended for fumigation.[5] At this concluding stage, a protective hymn specially addressed to Brahma should be chanted.

The above description is applicable for a planned operation. If the patient presents as an emergency with severe pain and distress, incision and drainage of the abscess should be done immediately "as a fire fighter puts out a fire."

Post-operative care:[6] After the hymn is chanted at the conclusion of the operation, the patient is shifted to his room. The standard graduated regimen for diet should be instituted and the bandage is changed on the third day; in summer and rainy weather, the dressing should be changed earlier on the second day. Suitable decoctions, local applications of ointments, and protection by bandages are carried out regularly in keeping with the season, time, and strength of the patient. No attempt should be made to speed up healing when any pus remains within. Healing should be promoted when the wound is clean.[7]

Basic surgical Procedures[8]

Basic surgical procedures stand in relation to surgical operations as words to sentences. There can be no sentences without words and words alone are infrequently used. One must learn the technique of doing basic procedures safely and well before attempting to do surgical operations such as plastic reconstruction of the nose or couching for cataract. Suśruta described eight basic procedures and used experimental methods to train students in performing them.

Basic procedures:

- Excision (chedya);
- Incision (bhedya);
- Scraping (lekhya);
- Puncture (vedhya);
- Probing (eṣya);
- Extraction (āhārya);
- Drainage/evacuation (visrāvya); and
- Suturing (sīvya)

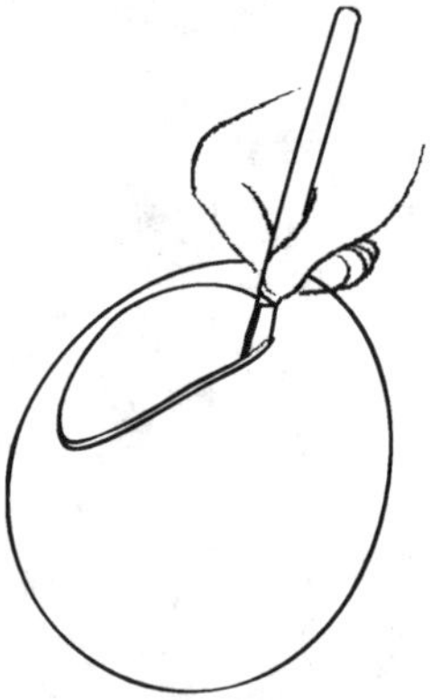

i. Excision (chedya) by excising a piece from a fruit with knife

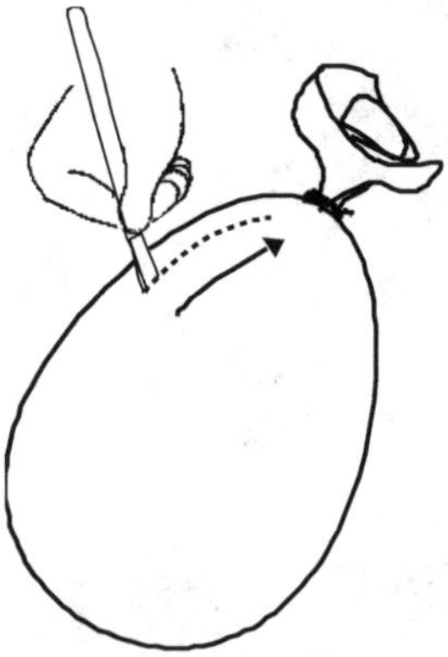

ii. Incision (Bhedya) by placing incision with a knife on a full leather bag

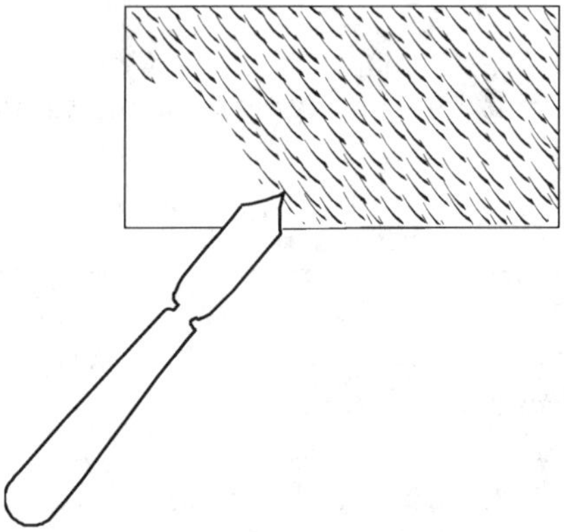

iii. Scraping (Lekhya) by scraping hair and hair follicles off by a special knife with two edges.

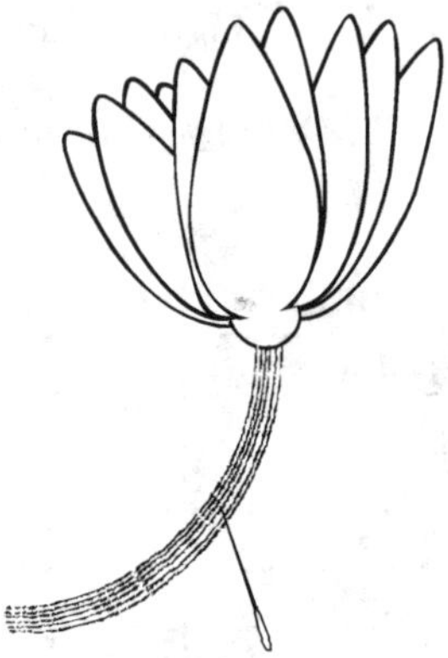

iv. Puncture (Vedhya) by puncturing on a lotus stalk with a needle

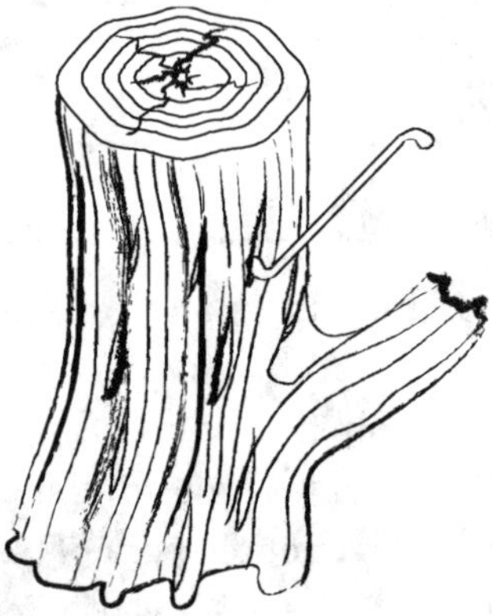

v. Probing (Eṣya) by probing a moth-eaten wood with metal probe

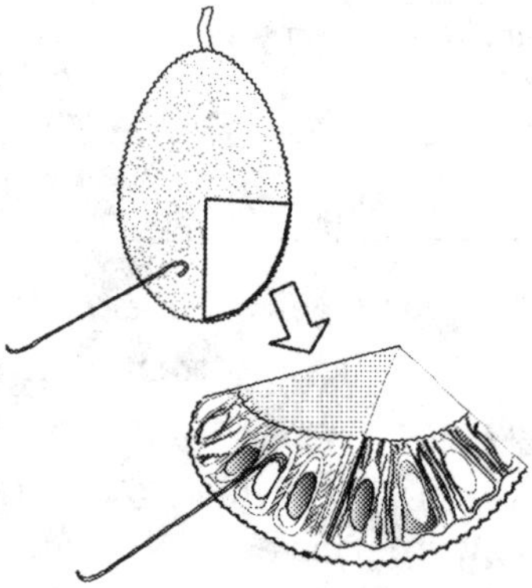

vi. Extraction (Āhārya) by using a probe with a hooked tip

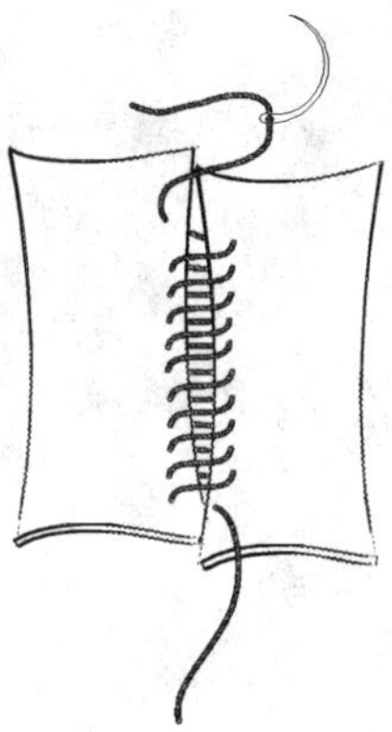

vii. Suturing (Sīvya) by sewing two pieces of thick cloth or leather by using curved needle and thread

Figure 2: Basic Surgical Procedures (i to vii)

The extensive use of basic procedures in different and commonly done operations is illustrated in Table 1.

Table 1: Examples of Basic Procedures employed in operations

Basic Procedures	Surgical operations
Excision (chedya)	Anal fistula, black mole, piles
Incision (bhedya)	Carbuncle, dental abscess, soft glandular swellings
Scraping (lekhya)	Vitiligo, ulcer tracks, scar
Puncture (vedhya)	Removing fluid from abdomen; scrotum; body channels
Probing (eṣya)	Sinus tracks to trace the cause: foreign bodies
Extraction (Āhārya)	• Gravel from urinary tract • Tartar of teeth • Ear wax
Drainage/Evacuation (visrāvya)	• Localised abscess • Inflamed ear lobe • Cystic swellings
Suturing (sīvya)	• Repair wounds caused by incision • Repair of fresh, clean wounds

Bandages: Bandages are essential to protect wound dressing and to immobilize body parts during the treatment of fractures and dislocations. Special types of bandages are necessary for application over joints, hips, moving parts such as chest, and organs such as eye and ear. Suśruta described 14 types of bandages of cloth made from linseed fibre, cotton, wool, silk, inner layer of the bark of trees, and animal skin. The technique for applying the bandage, "without folds or gaps in the desired pattern" was also described. The following figures illustrate some of the bandages described by Suśruta (Figure 3).

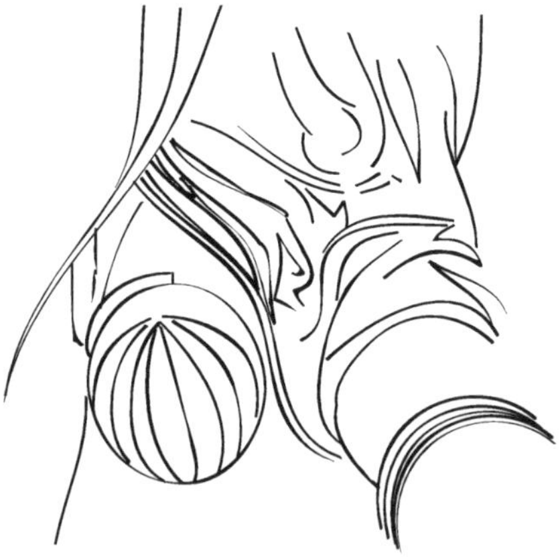

i. Sheath bandage for amputated limb (kośa)

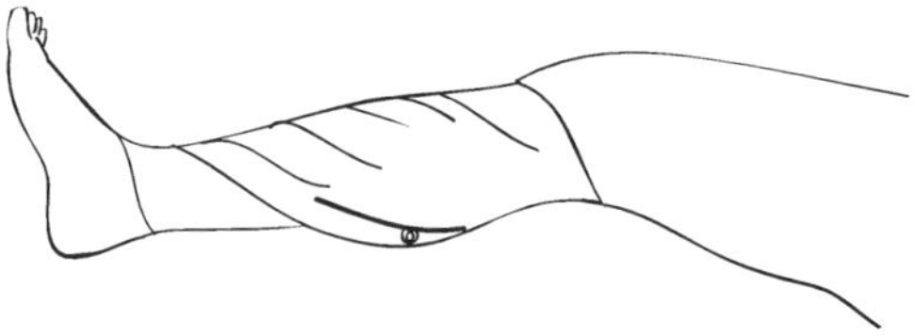

ii. Long roll for limbs (dāma)

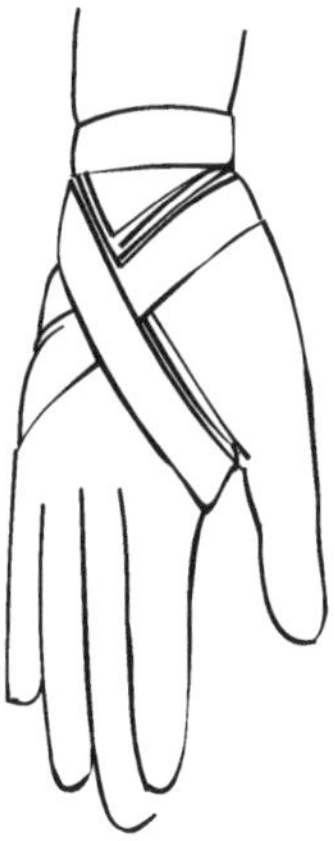

iii. Cross like (svastika) for palm

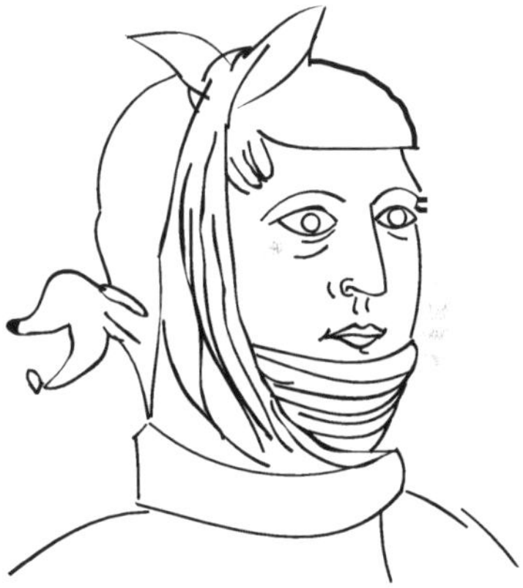

iv. Four-tailed (khaṭvā) for head and neck

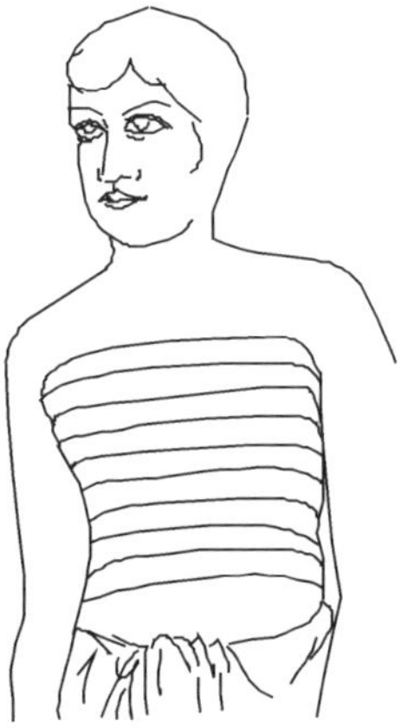

v. Circular (vibandha) for fracture ribs with moving chest

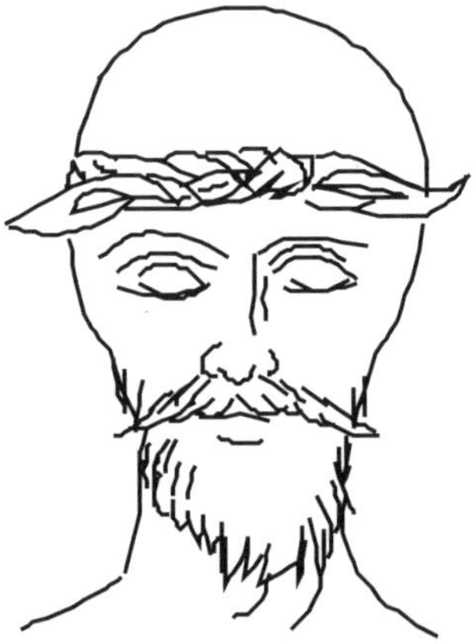

vi. Canopy like (vitāna) for protecting scalp wounds

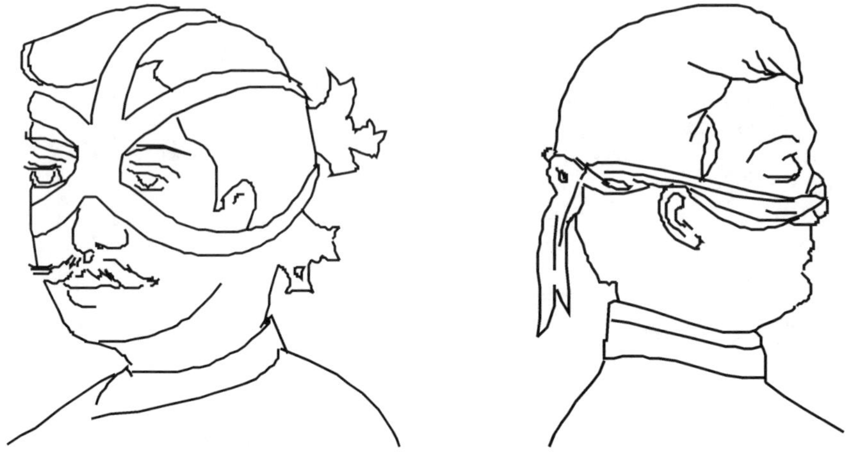

vii. String (goṣphaṇā) for nasal repair; often mentioned.

viii. Five-tailed (pañcāṅgī); for nasal and facial injuries.

Figure 3: Bandages (i to viii)

The descriptions were detailed and they specified the tightness of the bandage vis-à-vis the part or joint and the status of the injury; it was noted, "a tight bandage when medium or loose application is appropriate would squeeze out the medicated paste; if too loose instead of being tight, the paste laden wick would fall out, and bandage would rub on the wound."[9] If bandages are not used, the wounds would attract flies and medicinal pastes would dry up and lose their potency. Bandages protect wound, provide some degree of immobilization to the injured part, and enable the patient to move about and sleep well.[10]

Suśruta, however, recommended "open treatment" without bandage for wounds with severe pittaja features such as swelling, severe pain, discharge of pus, diabetic abscess, leprotic ulcers, and infections following rat bite.[11]

Errors in techniques: A conscious patient restrained in a surgical position by strong attendants, less than accurate knowledge of regional anatomy, the risk of punishment for serious errors, and above all, the pressure of time would unnerve most surgeons as they make the skin incision. Suśruta mentions a few errors made by surgeons such as too small, too large, or inappropriately placed incisions, and accidental injuries inflicted by the surgeon on his own hand. He attributed such errors to ignorance, confusion, fear, and surprisingly, greed! Surgeons responsible for such errors and the careless use of instruments, caustics, and cautery should be shunned by the public "like snakes."[12]

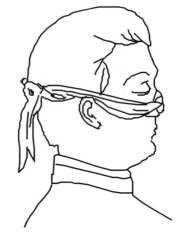

Surgical complications: Complications can be manifold following surgery. Injury of vital spots may be attended by collapse, bleeding, loss of consciousness, paralysis of limbs, and impaired sensations. Injury of major vessels would be followed by the gush of bright red blood: tendons by flaccidity, inability to move and poor healing; of joints by severe pain, large swelling, and immobility; of bone by pain day and night, severe thirst and immobility; there are similarly grave complications caused by injury to muscle. Oblique and extended incisions predispose to many of these complications and should be avoided as far as possible.

A fraudulent physician or a quack is murderous in his practice. On the contrary, a good physician is like a beneficent father whom the patient would trust implicitly and place himself in his care even if he lacks trust in his mother, father, sons, and relatives. By giving service with competence and good will, a surgeon gains virtue, prosperity, fame, friendship of the best, and a place in heaven in good time.[13]

Surgical Instruments

Suśruta's instruments constitute a jewel in the crown of India's surgical history. In the range of applications, workmanship, aesthetics, and directions on their expert use in the operating room, the instruments call out for recognition as a triumph of innovation and technology. It is obvious that surgical instruments, as refined and as diverse as in Suśruta's armamentarium, clould not be developed except as a collaborative effort of innovative surgeons, competent metal craftsmen, and the resources of ferrous metallurgy. It follows that this combination did exist in India in Suśruta's time because, he stipulates that the instruments must be made by skilled craftsmen (karma kovida). We shall have more to say about the technology of surgical instruments later.

Classification of instruments: Suśruta divided his instruments into two categories, blunt (yantras) and sharp (śastras). The blunt instruments were 100 in number and they were used for all kinds of applications except cutting. He pointed out however that among the blunt instruments, the foremost was the surgeon's hand without which other instruments would be useless and no procedure could be done in its absence! An abridged version of the blunt category of instruments is presented in Table 2.[14]

Table 2: Blunt Instruments (Yantras)

Examples (Named after animals) for removal of foreign bodies		
Types	Subtypes	Functions
Forceps (Svastika)	Sub types A (10) Examples: i. Lion forceps (simhamukha) ii. Tiger forceps (vyāghramukha) iii. Wolf forceps (vṛkamukha)	18 angulas long; two arms cross at a joint in the center: mouth shaped like that of wild animals; used for removing impacted foreign bodies(One angula 2.5 cm)
Forceps (Svastika)	Sub type B (15): Examples: i. Crow forceps (kākamukha) ii. Heron forceps (kaṅkamukha) iii. Osprey forceps (kurāramukha)	Design cruciform like subtype A; mouth shaped like birds; designed to fish out deep seated foreign bodies
Pincher forceps (Sandaṃśa)	i. With arms ii. Without arms	Design cruciform with two arms joined in the middle for depilation Two blades soldered at one end; to remove deep seated slough
Spoon-shaped instrument (Tālayantra)	i. Single blade (ekatāla) ii. Double blade (dvitāla)	Tip shaped like a spoon; to remove ear-wax: foreign bodies from nose, ear, etc.
Tubular Instruments (Nādīyantra)	11 types - Examples: i. Proctoscope (anal fistula) ii. Rectal cannula for enema	Open at one or both ends; used as endoscopes for visualisation; for drainage of fluids or removal of foreign bodies
Rod like instruments (Śalāka)	12 types - Examples: i. Snake hood-like (sarpaphaṇamukha) ii. Fish-hook like (baḍiśamukha)	Solid probes with tips designed for different applications
Instruments for venesection	i. Horn (śṛṅga) for cupping ii. Gourd (alābu)	

Figures 4 – 10 illustrate some of the instruments grouped under the blunt category.

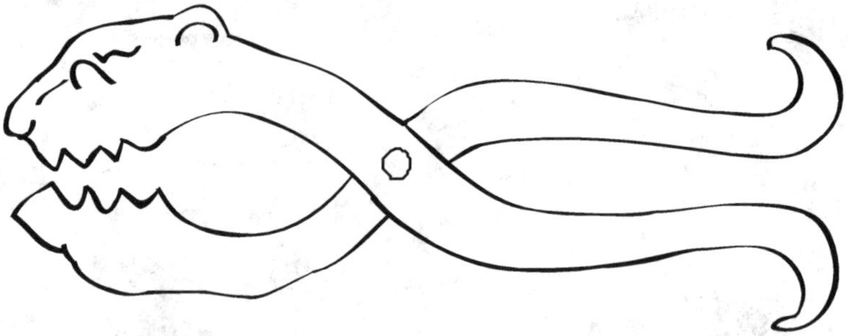

i. Lion face (simhamukha)

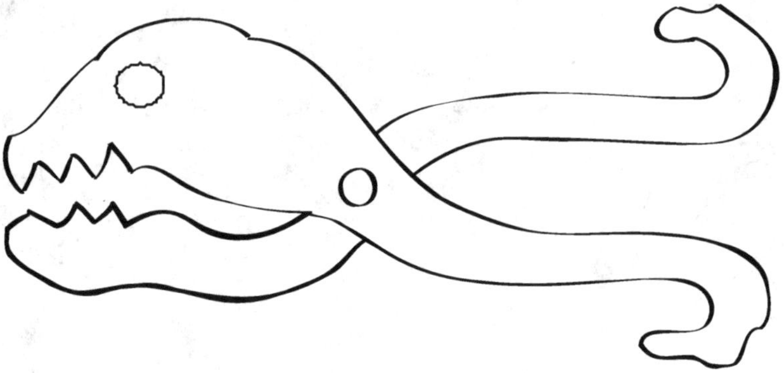

ii. Tiger face (vyāghramukha)

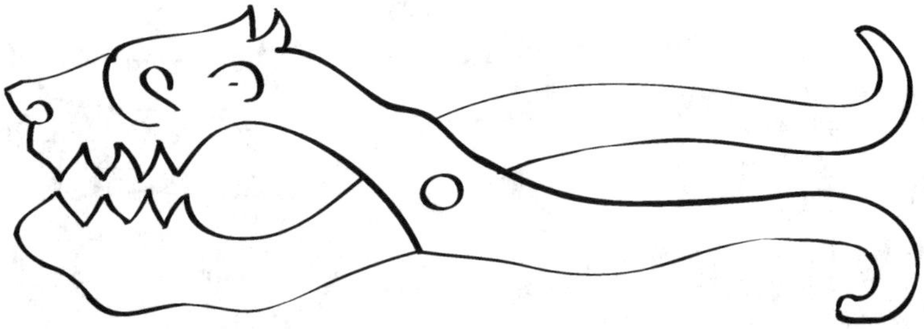

iii. Wolf face (vṛkamukha)

Figure 4: Forceps (Svastika)

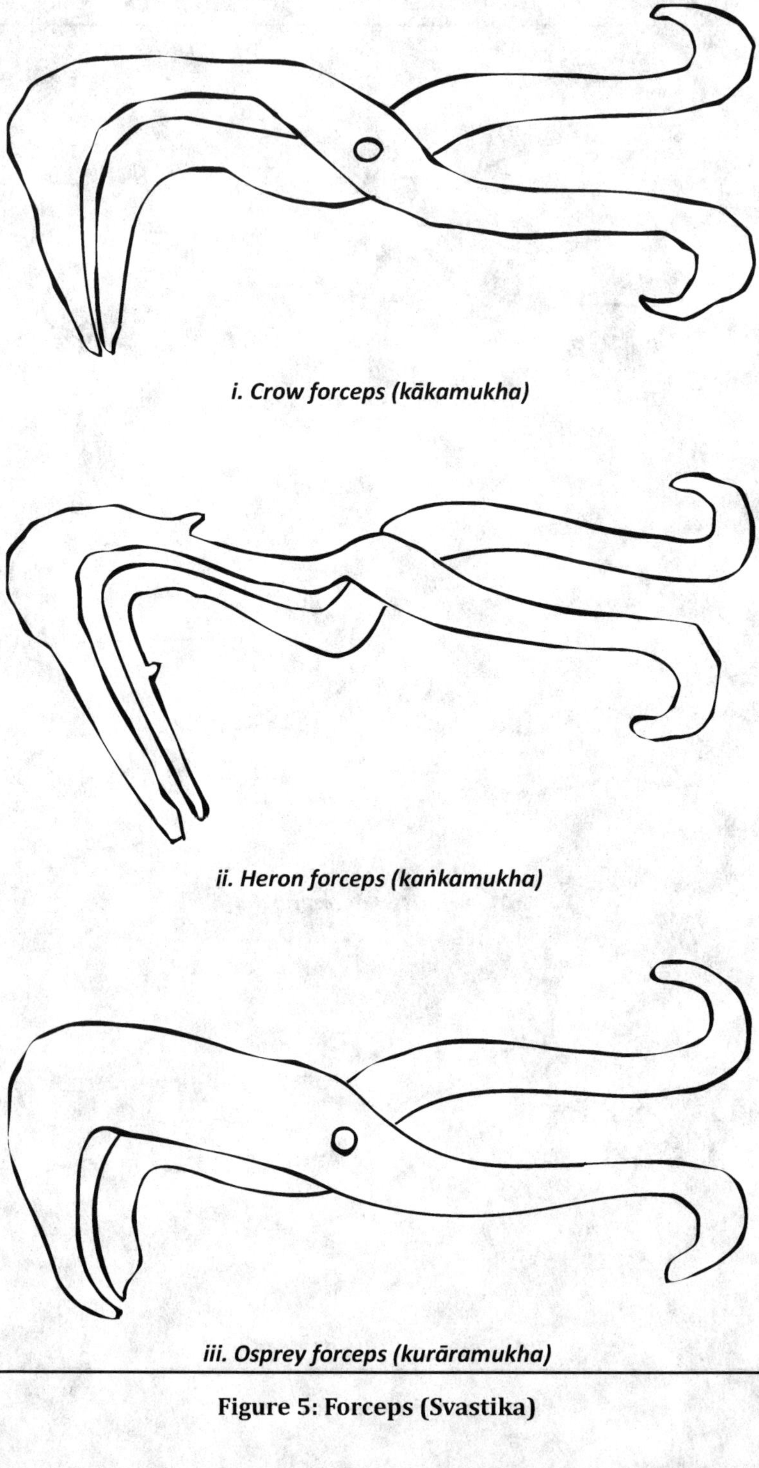

i. Crow forceps (kākamukha)

ii. Heron forceps (kaṅkamukha)

iii. Osprey forceps (kurāramukha)

Figure 5: Forceps (Svastika)

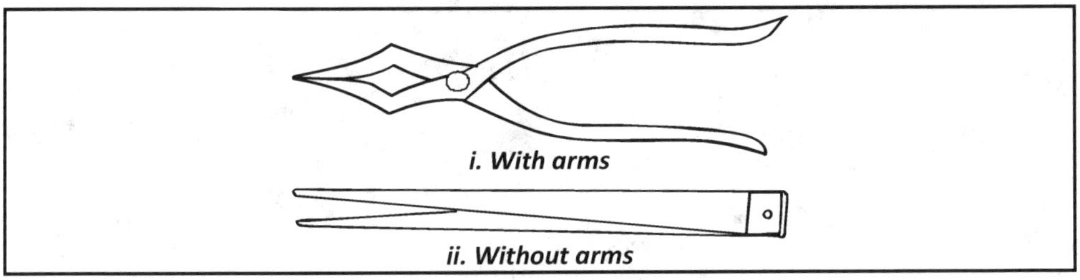

Figure 6: Pincher forceps (Sandaṃśa)

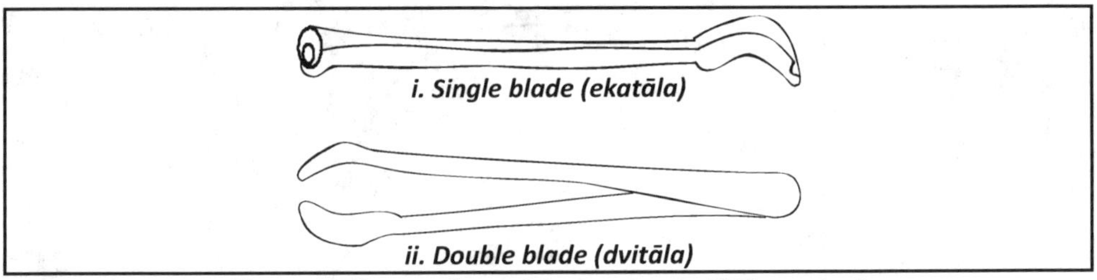

Figure 7: Spoon-shaped Instruments (Tālayantra)

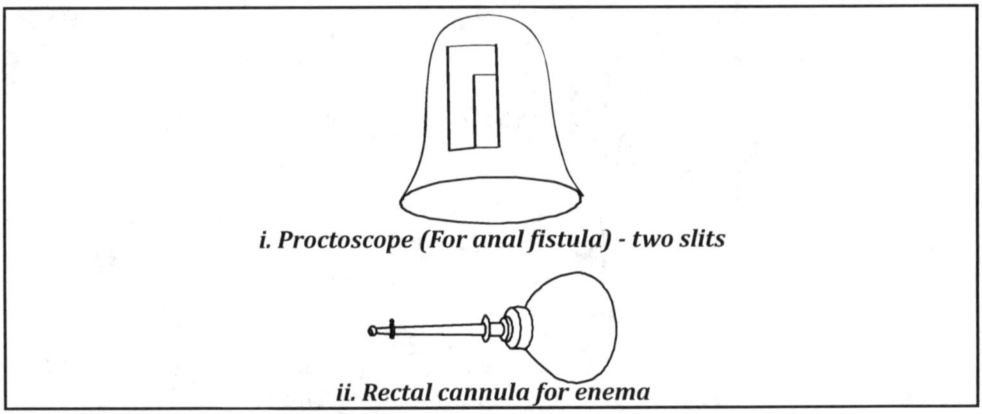

Figure 8: Tubular Instruments (Nāḍī Yantras)

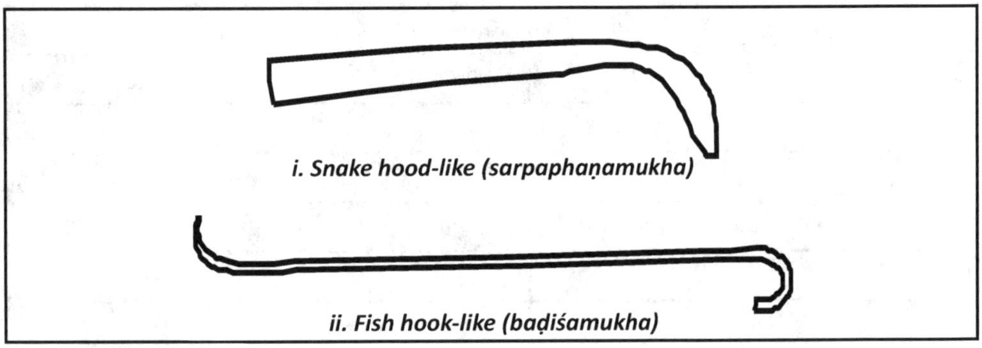

Figure 9: Rod-like Instruments (Śalāka)

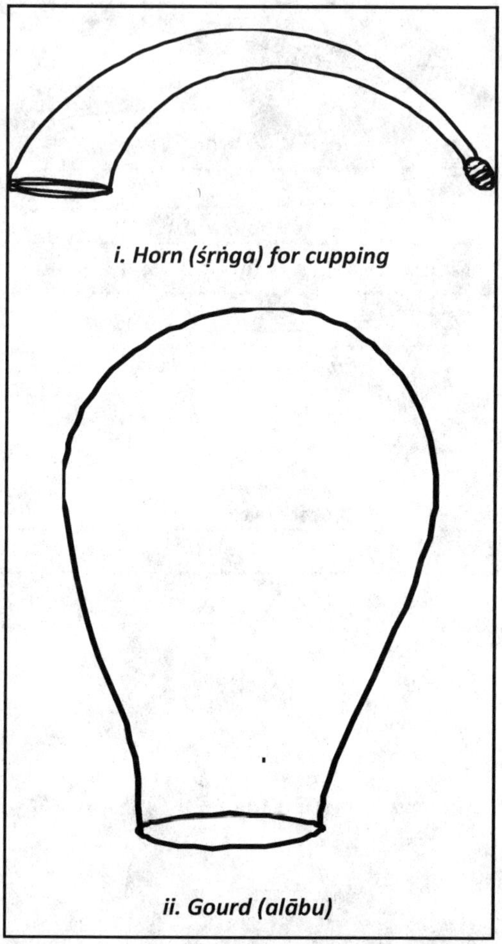

Figure 10: Instruments for venesection

Table 3: Sharp Instruments (śastras)15 – 20: Examples

Types	Comments
Maṇḍalāgra	Round tipped; for incision and scraping
Utpalapatra	Phlebotome
Karapatra	Serrated edge on one side
Vṛddhipatra	Straight-tipped scalpel
Śarārimukha	Scissors
Sūcī	Straight and curved

The above examples are illustrated in Figure 11.

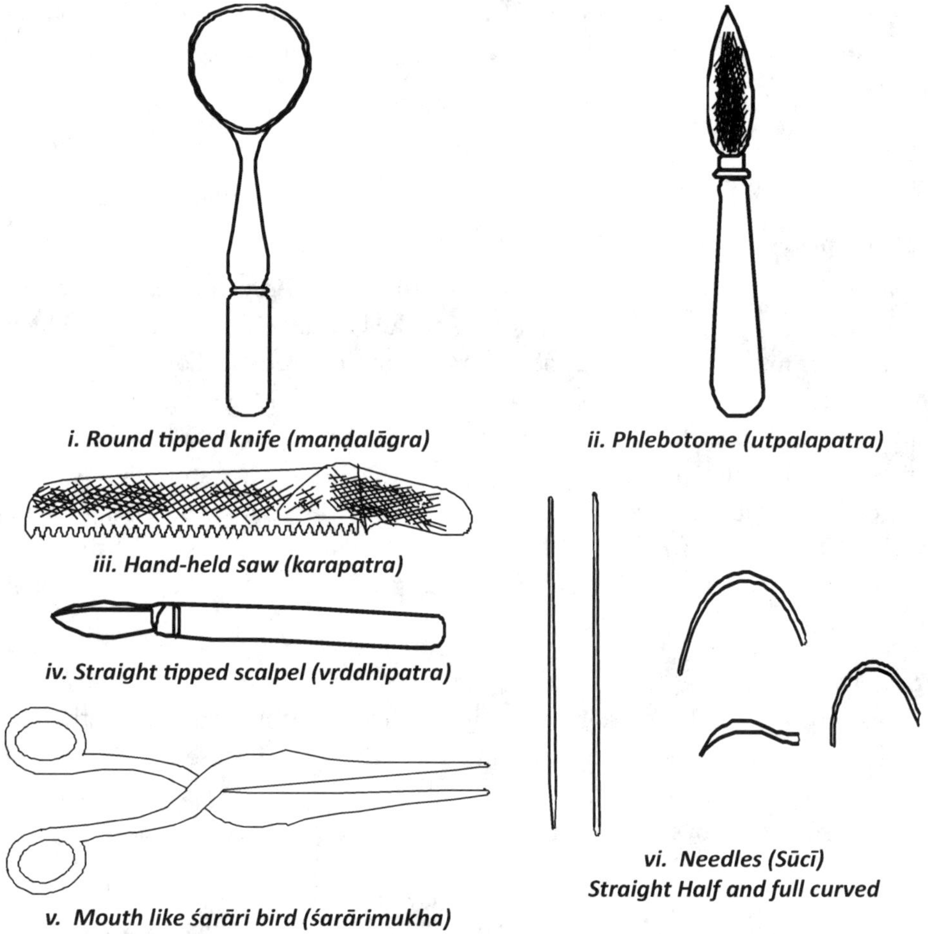

Figure 11: Sharp Instruments (śastras)

Table 4: Accessory Instruments (Upayantras)–25: Examples:

i. Thread (rajju) ii. Bandages (patta) iii. Leather	iv. Tree bark v. Cloth vi. Hammer vii. Nail	viii. Caustic ix. Cautery x. Medications

Sharp Instruments (20) were the "cutting edge" of Śalya. Some of them are illustrated in Figures 10 and 11.

Handling of Instruments: Instruments should be checked for defects such as too long, too short, broken tips, too hard to hold, cracks, etc., before use. The instrument chosen should be the most appropriate for the application. A sharp instrument, well designed, well made, sharp enough to divide hair, and easy to handle alone should be used in operations. The handling of instruments during operations is an art with economy in hand movement. The cleaning and proper storage of instruments should be done after every procedure.[16]

As the success of a surgeon depends on the skillful use of instruments, he should practice on them continuously.[17]

Associated procedures: Caustics; Cautery: Blood letting

For a patient and his family, surgery would be the last option. They would always prefer medical treatment; if that does not work, they would opt for a method which would be more invasive than medical treatment but less drastic than surgery. The three procedures listed above – caustics, cautery, and bloodletting – fall within this intermediate zone. By tacitly agreeing to this graded approach to a surgical option, Suśruta had anticipated John Hunter of the 18th century and celebrated as the pioneer of surgical science. Hunter said, "Now, the last part of surgery, namely operations, is a reflection on the healing art. It is a tacit admission of the inadequacy of surgery. It is like an armed savage trying to get by force what a civilized man would get by stratagem."

Caustics (Kṣāra):[18] The term kṣāra means the preparation of alkalis for clinical use and also the procedure (kṣāra karma) for its application. It is a reputed method in so far as it addresses not only the local manifestation of a disease but also of the underlying disturbance of doṣas. It combines multiple roles of excision, incision, scarification, and employs several drugs. It is "agneya" (fiery) by nature.

Kṣāra may be used as a paste for local application or given orally as a drug. The paste is applied for treating a variety of conditions such as skin diseases including leprosy, anal fistula, tumours, piles, vitiated ulcers, warts, sinuses on the skin, abscess, worms, and moles.[19] The ingestible form of kṣāra is given for the treatment of many disease conditions including the consumption of man-made poisons, gaseous lumps of the abdomen (gulma), poor appetite, indigestion, constipation, worms, and piles.[20] It is contra-indicated in internal bleeding, fever, paittika disorders, children, elderly, and emaciated persons.

Suśruta gave an excellent description of the preparation of a kṣāra from a muṣkaka tree, starting with the sacred ritual for cutting the tree to the elaborate process involving a number of other plants, and several steps in production. The method of preparing kṣāra of high, medium, and low strength was also specified.[21]

To apply the kṣāra paste, the procedure room was made ready just as for a surgical operation. The diseased area was cleaned, gently rubbed, and scarified before kṣāra was applied and kept in place for one hundred mātras (a mātra is the time to pronounce a short syllable). As soon as the surface shows blackening and fragmentation, a mixture of sour substances, ghee, and madhuka should be applied to neutralize the kṣāra. If the surface does not readily separate, another application of a neutralizing paste should be done, which usually works and promotes wound healing. When done properly, the disease settles and the part feels light. The prohibition of kṣāra on various types of individuals, parts of the body, and clinical conditions should be carefully noted before its application.[22]

Cauterisation (Agni karma): Cauterisation ranks higher than caustics in rooting out disease and may work better than caustics in treating diseases resistant to drugs. Generally, cauterisation is confined to skin but, according to Suśruta, it can also be done to deeper structures including blood vessels, tendons, and joints.[23] It can be done in all seasons except autumn and summer, but in emergencies any season is suitable for intervention.

In performing cauterisation, the important considerations are the location and area of the disease and how a vital spot close by could be saved, strength of the patient, and the season. Suśruta provides a list of conditions affecting skin, muscle, blood vessels, tendon, bone and joints, anal fistula, wart, elephantiasis etc., which are suitable for cauterisation. Diseases of forehead and eyelids are also considered favourably for cauterisation. A large number of contra-indications are also given.[24]

Burns and treatment: The section on cauterisation also includes a short discussion on burns. Burns are classified with four grades depending on their depth as follows:[25]

1. Pluṣṭa: Loss of normal colour, no vesicles, charring;
2. Durdagdha: Severe pain, burning, redness, blisters;
3. Samyakdagdha: Superficial, colour of ripe dates, no blisters; and
4. Atidagdha: Flesh exposed and hangs loose, injured vessels, tendons, joints, bones, severe pain.

The four types are treated as outlined below:

Burns grade	**Principles treatment**
Pluṣṭa	Warm fomentation; diet and drugs to raise body heat
Durdagdha	Apply ghee locally; medicated paste and irrigation with cold water or decoctions
Samyakdagdha	Warm paste of vegetable or animal products applied
Atidagdha	Excision of slough; cold applications of paste of vegetable products such as śali rice or tinḍuki bark ground in ghee. Treat like pittaja cellulitis.

Suśruta also briefly refers to inhalation injury by smoke[26] and its management by emesis, hydration, nasal purging, light, and greasy diet. It makes one wonder about forest fires and forest dwellers being carried to Suśruta's ashram in dire conditions, overwhelmed by smoke!

Bloodletting (Rakta visrāvaṇa)

Bloodletting was used extensively in Āyurveda for treating a variety of ailments such as skin disorders, glandular swellings, and diseases of blood. In surgery, it constitutes nearly half of clinical management and has a position equivalent to that of enema in medical treatment.[27] Patients with inflammatory disease of recent onset, fixed chronic ulcers with irregular margins, and squelae of snake bite are especially suitable for bloodletting. It is forbidden in patients with emaciation, pallor, dropsy, phthisis, and pregnant women.

The two methods used for bloodletting are scarification and venesection. In scarification, a series of skin-deep scratches are made with a sharp instrument sparing vital spots, blood vessels, and joints. The season, timing of the procedure, and technique are important in making the scarification procedure effective. Methods to enhance blood flow or arrest the blood flow from the wound and management of the patient after the procedure were described.[28] A successful procedure is marked by spontaneous arrest of bleeding, feeling of lightness, relief from pain, reduced intensity of illness, and cheerfulness.[29]

Venesection was used widely and the contra-indications were similar to those for scarification. The patient was prepared by lubricant therapy and fomentation and given a liquid diet with qualities opposed to those of his perturbed doṣas. The selected part of the body was kept immobilized by tying it just tight enough to make the veins prominent. The positioning of the patient and application of a tourniquet for different veins was clearly described. A skin incision of "the depth of a barley grain" was made over the prominent vein which was opened with a special knife. The blood which flows out is vitiated; blood flow may diminish or stop if the patient is fearful or dehydrated. If necessary, the procedure can be repeated on the same day. It is preferable to leave behind some vitiated blood and treat the remainder left behind by medical therapy. The maximum permissible limit for bloodletting is 648 ml.[30] The conditions for which venesection used for treatment were many and varied.[31]

In addition to scarification and venesection, horn, gourd, and leeches were also used for bloodletting. All methods seek to remove vitiated blood from the patient's body. Generally, leeches are used for deep seated illness, scarification when the disease is localised, horn and gourd for skin disorders, and venesection for generalized vitiation of blood of the whole body.

Leeches (Jalaukā): Leeches were used from ancient times for bloodletting. In the Atharvaveda, "leech" was used as a synonym for a physician. It was lauded as an instrument in the hand of Lord Dhanvantari in the first line of his memorable invocation:

ॐशंखंचक्रंजलौकांदधिदमृतघटंचारुदोर्भिश्चतुर्भिः।
[Glory to Lord Dhanvantari, cradling conch, discus, leech and pot of nectar in his beneficent four hands]

Leeches were considered the gentlest method for bloodletting, suitable for kings, children, elderly, timid and weak persons, and women. Twelve types of leeches were described of which six are without poison.[32] The non-venomous types are plentiful in north west India and pāndya country and they are large, sturdy, quick to suck, and voracious. The catching and cultivation of leeches in-house were described with a view to therapeutic requirements.[33] The method of applying leeches for bloodletting, signs of satisfactory progress in sucking by the leech, how to deal with problems such as the leech failing to suck or patient complaining of pain, how to make the leech regurgitate the blood it had sucked and care of the wound were described in detail for the practicing physiciain.[34] It is interesting that bloodletting by phlebotomy was used in the 20th century for the treatment of cardiac and hematological conditions when the proportion of the cellular components of blood reached abnormal levels.

References

1. *SS Sūtra* 1: 16 – 19
2. Kauṭilya's *Arthaśāstra* Tr. Shama Satry, Mysore 1967. Page 233
3. *SS Sūtra*5: 6
4. *SS Sūtra*5: 11 – 15
5. *SS Sūtra*5: 16 - 18
6. *SS Sūtra*5: 34 – 39
7. *SS Sūtra*5: 41 - 42
8. *SS Sūtra*25: 3 – 19
9. *SS Sūtra*18: 24 - 26
10. *SS Sūtra*18: 20 – 30
11. *SS Sūtra*18: 31 – 34
12. *SS Sūtra*25: 30 – 33
13. *SS Sūtra*25: 41 – 45

14. *SS Sūtra*7: 10 – 15
15. *SS Sūtra* 8: 3 – 9, 14, 19
16. *SS Sūtra* 8: 12 – 13
17. *SS Sūtra* 8: 15 – 20
18. *SS Sūtra* 11: 3 – 5
19. *SS Sūtra* 11: 6 – 7
20. *SS Sūtra* 11: 8 – 9
21. *SS Sūtra* 11: 16 – 17
22. *SS Sūtra* 11: 18 – 29
23. *SS Sūtra* 12: 3 – 7
24. *SS Sūtra* 12: 8
25. *SS Sūtra* 12: 16
26. *SS Sūtra* 12: 29 - 32
27. *SS Sūtra* 8: 23
28. *SS Sūtra* 14: 35
29. *SS Sūtra* 14: 29 - 33
30. *SS Śārīra* 8: 9 - 16
31. *SS Śārīra* 8: 17
32. *SS Sūtra* 13: 9 - 10
33. *SS Sūtra* 13: 16 - 17
34. *SS Sūtra* 13: 19 - 22

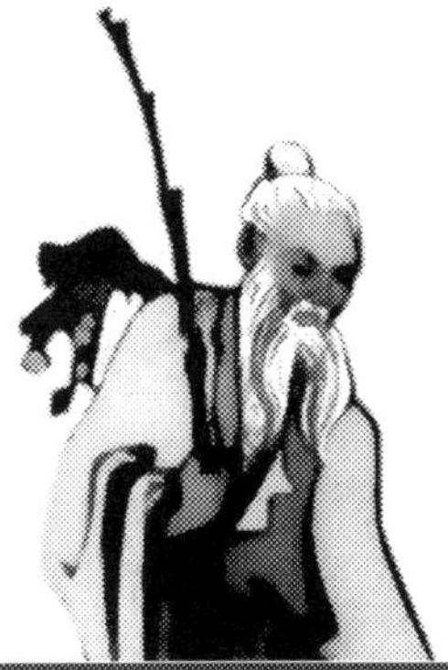

CHAPTER 13

Treatment of Fractures: Selected Surgical Procedures

The previous chapter being an overview of surgical treatment pioneered by Suśruta, the present chapter will focus on specific examples of procedures and surgical operations, which demonstrate the high standards of excellence attained by surgeons in ancient India.

Fractures:[1] Treatment of fractures is a good subject to begin with, as they were common in times of peace and war and Suśruta dealt with them exhaustively. He clearly distinguished fractures from dislocations and noted that fractures occurred due to fall from trees or bullock carts, falling of trees on individuals, and attacks by wild animals or combatants in wars. He classified fractures into 12 types, which have a contemporary ring. They are outlined below:

Table 1: Fractures

Type	Comments
1. Karkaṭaka	Mid shaft fracture of long bones of the limbs; fracture ends slightly at angle
2. Aśvakarṇa	Same as above; but the fractured ends at greater angle with greater deformity of the limbs
3. Cūrṇita	Comminuted fracture; fractured ends shattered
4. Picchita	Bone subjected to crush injury
5. Asthicalita	Two fractured ends displaced downwards and sideways with wide gap
6. Kāṇḍabhagna	Fractured ends move free due to lack of muscular attachment
7. Majjānugata	One fractured end impacted into the other end
8. Atipātita	One fractured end pulled up by muscle attachment; the other end droops
9. Vakra	Green stick (in children)
10. Chinna	One fractured end shattered, and the other end intact
11. Pāṭita	Number of penetrating holes on one side of bone with no complete through-and-through injury
12. Sphuṭita	Bone cracked; no displacement; "hair-line" fracture

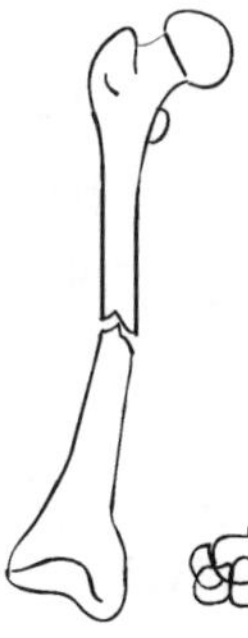

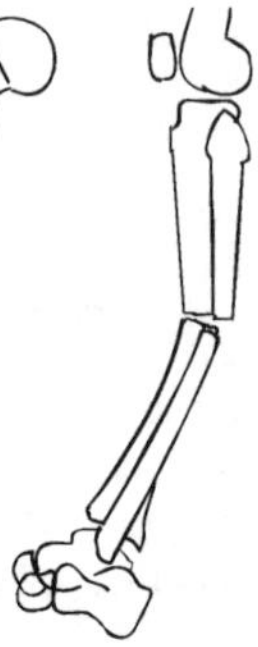

1. Karkaṭaka *2. Aśvakarṇa*

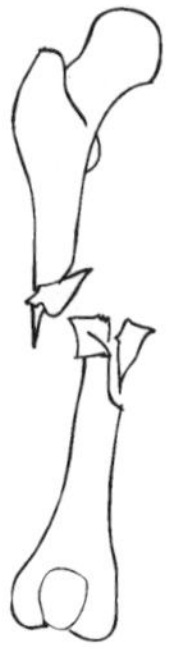

3. Cūrṇita

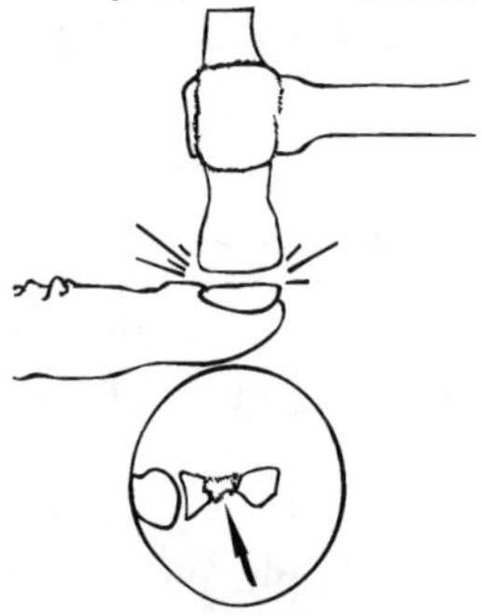

4. Picchita

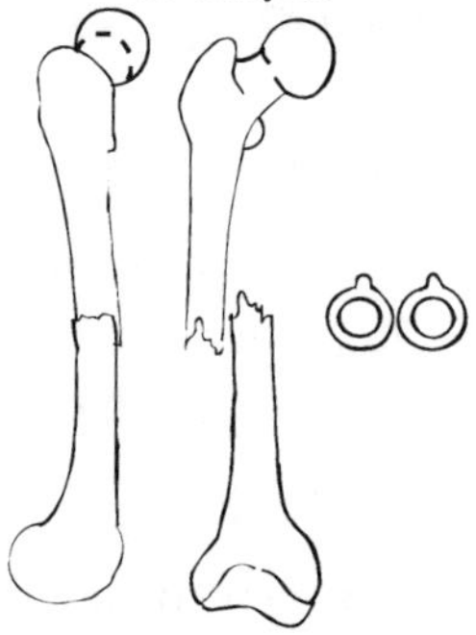

5. Asthicalita

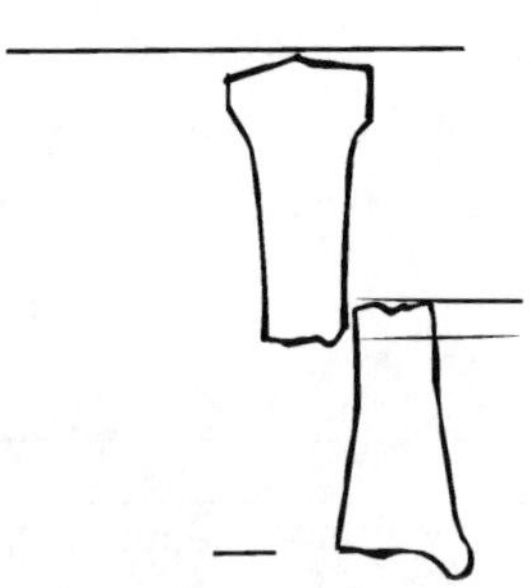

6. Kāṇḍabhagna

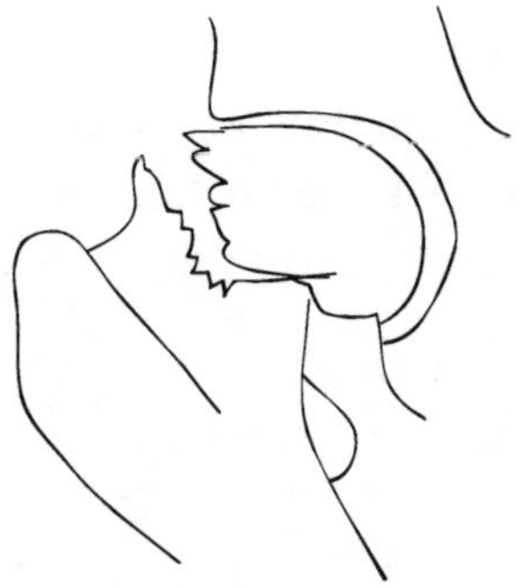

7. Majjānugata

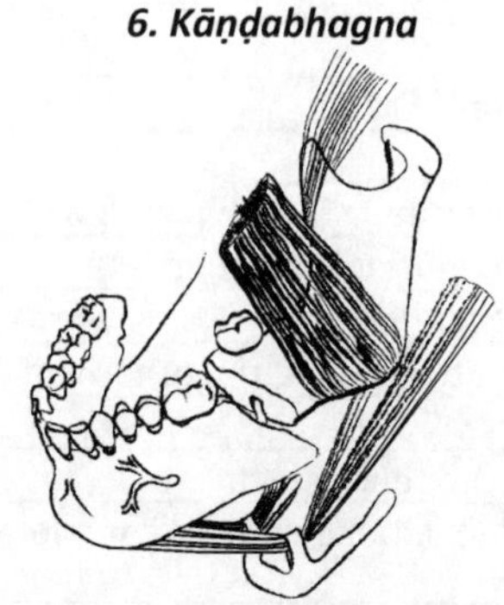

8. Atipātita

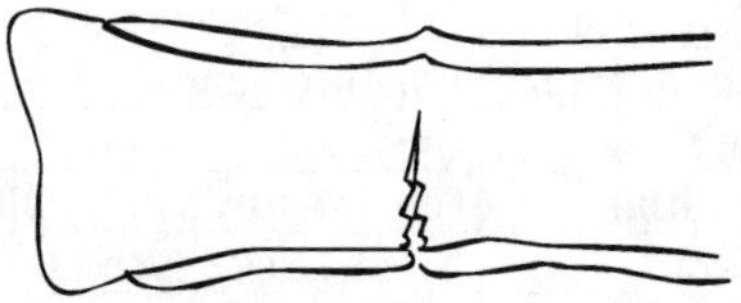

9. Vakra

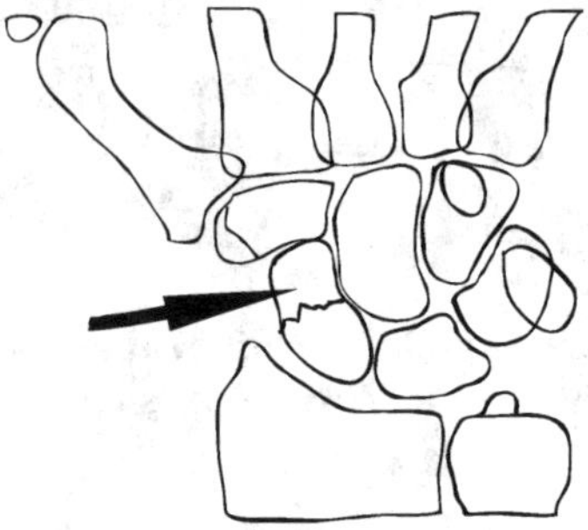

10. Sphuṭita

Figure 1–10: Fractures

It is important to remember that this classification was made in Suśruta's time, when no imaging of bones was even dreamt of! The classification was made possible by accurate observation, creative imagination, and years of experience.

Treatment of fractures

A great deal of attention was paid to general measures including nutritious diet, rest, wound toilet, suture, and applications of medical pastes whenever necessary.[2] The local measures, to reduce pain and promote healing of the fracture took priority. This involved four steps:[3]

- Traction (āñcana);
- Compression (pīdana);
- Immobilisation (saṃkṣepa); and
- Bandaging (bandhana),

Traction (āñcana): Traction of the distal part against counter-traction from the proximal part of the fracture would bring the two ends into alignment.

Compression (pīdana): Implied manipulation and repositioning of the fractured ends, both of which would include some degree of firm holding of the limb or compression. These manipulations could not be done without giving heavy doses of wine to the patient and his physical control.

Immobilisation (saṃkṣepa): This was done by the use of splints made of bamboo, bark of trees etc., and subsequent bandaging (Figure: 11). Immobilisation was done differently when the fracture involved the thigh bone (femur) or the long bone of the leg (tibia). In both cases, patients would not be able to walk or put weight on the affected leg. Here, the method employed was a fracture bed with a flat and rigid surface, where the patient would recline and his joints above and below the fracture would be immobilised by suitable placement of pegs as shown (Figure 12).

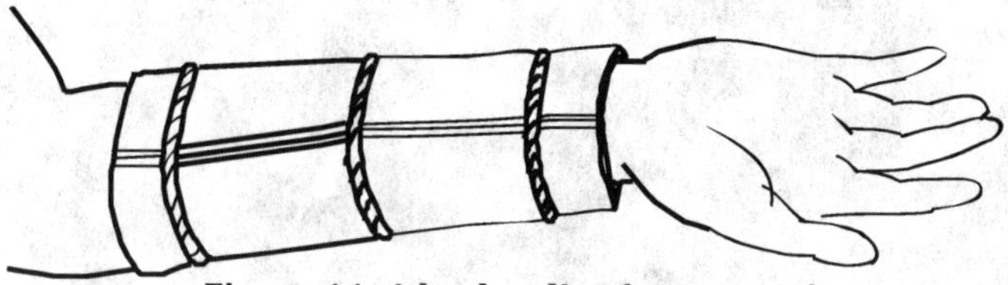

Figure 11: A bark splint (upayantra)
Bark splint is made from trees such as aśvattha

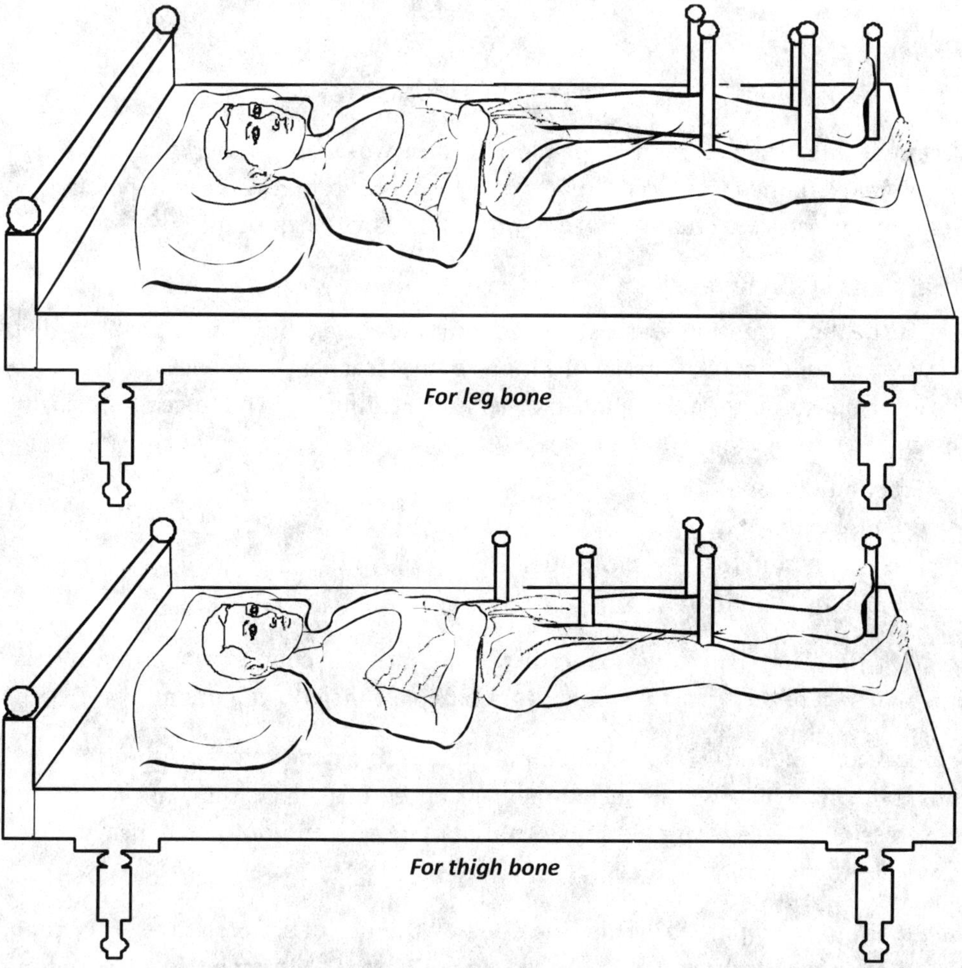

Figure 12: Fracture bed (kapāṭaśayana): Joints above and below immobilized by pegs; foot stabilized by single peg

Management of regional fractures would pose special problems and directions were given on the treatment of fracture of hand and foot, pelvis, ribs, shoulder, elbow, palms, collar bone, neck, jaw, teeth, nose, ear, and skull.[4]

If, the pelvis had sustained fracture with bone displacement, the prognosis was recognised to be so poor that the physician was advised to refrain from excessive attempts at treatment. Similar caution was advised when patients with serious injuries including fracture were badly treated elsewhere and ended up with a physician in dire condition.[5]

Medications: Suśruta Saṃhitā (SS) recommends a number of medicinal pastes, which cleanse the wounds in case of compound fractures and promote healing.[6] Herbal drugs are also prescribed specifically to promote fracture healing.[7] A good outcome of fracture treatment was adjudged from the absence of deformity, of lengthening or shortening of the extremity, comfort, and unrestricted movement.

Selected surgical procedures

As SS deals with a large number of surgical operations, it would serve our purpose to review a few representative samples, which cover specialties as we have already referred to a commonly done general surgical procedure of incision and drainage of abscess in the previous chapter (chapter 12). The specialized procedures chosen are the following:

- Plastic reconstruction of the nose
- Removal of foreign bodies
- Piles

Plastic reconstruction of nose: It is intriguing that this operation, which is arguably the most famous surgical operation to win global recognition as an original method developed in India is covered in five verses in SS, which devotes eight verses to describe incision and drainage of an abscess. A possible explanation for this anomaly could be that the plastic operation on the nose had already gone out of the main stream of Āyurveda and was no longer being done by physicians by the fourth century when SS was redacted by Nāgārjuna.

Suśruta's original technique involved taking a pedicled flap from the forehead of the patient, but the technique observed by British physicians in Pune consisted of a flap from the cheek. A tree leaf is cut exactly according to the defect in the nose, a pedicled flap of the skin is raised from the cheek as per the cut leaf, flap is placed on the nasal defect after freshening its edges, with pedicle still attached to the cheek, and flap is fixed in position with herbal glue (Figure 13). The nasal orifices are kept open under the flap with two tubes, which would keep the flap elevated. This is followed by spraying a powder of red sandalwood, madhūka, and rasāñjana on the wound, while cotton soaked in sesamum oil is used to dress the grafted flap. Medicated ghee is given to the patient, when he feels hungry indicating that his previous meal has been digested. A purgative should be administered subsequently as per usual protocol. When the flap has healed well, the base of the pedicle should be divided and the edges of the flap trimmed to give it a good cosmetic result.[8]

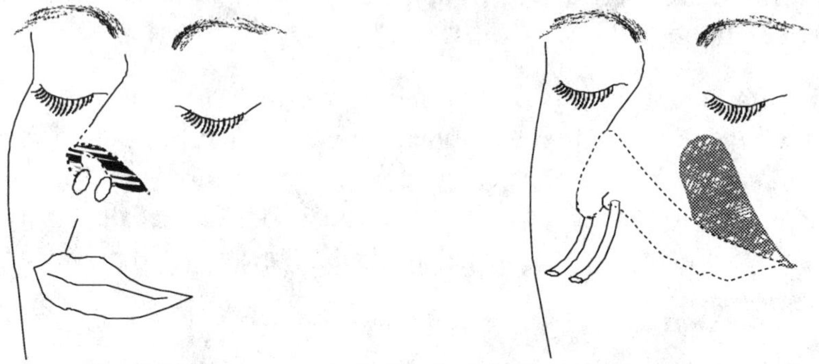

Nasal defect

Flap from adjacent cheek turned to reconstruct the nose. Note the tubes inserted to keep nasal orifices open.

Figure 13: Reconstruction of the nose

Foreign bodies and their removal: Foreign bodies embedded in body tissues were a major concern in ancient times. They are of two types viz., endogenous or produced within the body and exogenous or introduced from outside. The endogenous group includes teeth, hair, nails, necrotic tissue, and vitiated doṣas; all others are exogenous. Both types give rise to pain and other symptoms.[9] The exogenous bodies could be metals, wooden splinters, horns, and bones. Among the metallic variety, arrowheads are the most dangerous, especially the barbed ones. They may enter the body from different directions and stop at various depths. They could stop and lodge themselves in the skin or deeper in the vessels, muscle, bone, or marrow cavity.

The site of entry of a foreign body would be swollen with black discoloration, pain, and frothy and blood stained discharge. The site of lodgement of the body in the skin, muscle, veins, ligaments, arteries, bone, joints, and abdomen would produce characteristic clinical features, which would lead a physician to a diagnosis.[10] From a prognostic angle, if the point of entry of the foreign body is in the line of direction of hair, the wound would heal, especially in areas like neck, veins, muscle, and marrow cavity. Migration of foreign bodies would increase the risk for the patient.

Detection of deeply embedded foreign bodies, which are not visible, would call for special measures for their location. This involves oil application on the part, massage with powdered earth, māṣa, barley, wheat, and cow dung, when the site of the lodgement of the foreign body would throw up signs of inflammation. Variations of this technique may be used for locating the foreign bodies lodged in the veins, bones, and body cavities at greater depth.

Sometimes, the test for localization would involve riding in a chariot with broken wheels, or on the nape of an elephant or on the back of a horse, practice of wrestling, long jump or high jump – all directed to shaking up the implanted foreign body at a depth. These signs may be aided by patient's complaints of "pins and needles," local loss of sensation, heaviness, swelling, severe pain, and tendency to guard a spot. If the wound shows tendency to heal with significant reduction in symptoms, the track of the foreign body should be thoroughly explored with a suitable probe and unhindered movement of adjacent joints ensured before excluding the presence of a foreign body. The foreign bodies are known to bend or break; if they are wooden in origin and not extracted, they will cause suppuration and vitiation of blood. If they are made of gold, silver, copper, brass, tin, or lead, they may, over a long period, get incorporated in body tissues through the working of pitta. However, objects made of horn, tooth, hair, bone, stone, bamboo, and earth do not disintegrate and disappear.[11]

Extraction of foreign bodies: From the point of view of the removal of foreign bodies, they belong to the loose or fixed categories. The loose category gets removed by 15 measures. Examples:

- **Spontaneous elimination:** Lachrymation, sneezing, coughing, micturition, defecation etc., depending on location.
- **Suppuration:** It may be spontaneous or could be induced by fomentation etc. The foreign body passes out with the pus.
- **Incision and drainage of abscess:** The Foreign body is eliminated through pus.
- **Wiping off:** E.g.: The Eye
- **Air and food passages:** Forced expiration, cough, or emesis induced by drugs or tickling of the throat could expel foreign bodies.
- **Irrigation, suction, sucking, and magnet:** Applicable for removal of objects from ulcers; for vitiated blood, breast milk; for iron–based foreign body in a wide mouth cavity.[12]

Techniques of surgical removal of foreign bodies:

❖ Surgical removal may be done in the direction in which the object made its entry (anuloma), or it may be done in the opposite direction (pratiloma). The pratiloma technique is used when the object has penetrated less than half the depth of the body part (e.g.: the leg); anuloma is applied when the penetration extends more than half of the depth.

- If a cutting edge is sticking out and is visible, it should be cut out and the object removed by manipulation after firmly holding it with forceps.
- If the location is in a body cavity like abdomen or chest, effort should be made for manipulation and removal by hand; if that fails, the track should be widened or extended by a cutting instrument and the foreign body pulled out by forceps. If surgery is done, the wound should be treated with standard techniques including haemostasis, cauterisation, fomentation, application of medicinal pastes, and bandaging.[13]

  When a foreign body is implanted in a bone, it should be gripped firmly by forceps and pulled out, while counter traction is exerted by the surgeon's foot on the patient's body. There are also adventurous techniques, such as the visible part of the foreign body being tied to one end of a bow string and the other end being tied to the rein of a horse with a bandage. As soon as the horse is whipped, it would lift its head forcefully and pull out the foreign body in that process.[14]

Foreign body in the throat: When an object like a fish bone gets stuck in the throat and blocks the air and food passages, it could be an emergency. It was recommended that a hair ball (keśondukam) with a string attached should be swallowed by the patient with sips of thin gruel until his stomach was full. He should then be made to vomit, when the string would enmesh itself in the foreign body. At that moment, the string should be pulled out with the foreign body. If the patient develops sores in the throat, they should be treated with the pastes of honey and ghee. When a food bolus blocks the throat, a sudden blow by the fist on the back of the neck may serve to dislodge it.

The wise surgeon should understand the nature of the foreign body lodged within the body, in terms of its size, structure (feathered, barbed etc.), and plan to extract them with the most appropriate instruments.[15]

Piles: Piles was a common ailment and received a great deal of attention in Ayurvedic classics. Suśruta classified piles into six types, which were caused by perturbation of vāta, pitta, kapha, blood, a combination of all four, and lastly, heredity. The cause of non-hereditary types was attributed to over eating, dietary indiscretion, incompatible food, sexual excess, prolonged squatting position, riding on animal's back, and suppression of physical urges. The perturbed doṣas reach the rectum through large vessels (pradhāna dhamani) and produce fleshy protrusions, which slowly increase in size. These are piles.[16]

According to Suśruta, anorectum (guda) measures four and half fingers in length and begins at the end of the large bowel. It has three sphincters or folds within (valaya), at intervals of one and half fingers each known as pravahaṇī, visarjanī, and samvaraṇī (Figure 14). The anal verge is one and half "yava" from the hairline. The first fold is one finger away from the anal verge.[17]

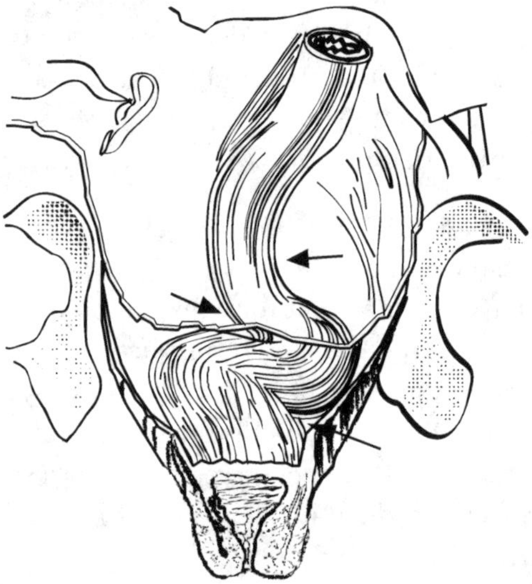

Figure 14: Rectum; folds and chambers; arrows point to the folds and change in the direction of flow.

The prodromal features of piles include loss of appetite, acid eructations, abdominal fullness, recurrent belching, audible bowel sounds, cough, drowsiness, and malaise. When piles related local features appear, vātika type is dry, reddish resembling Kadamba flowers and may have a tubular or bud like presentation with painful defecation, pain in the perineum, rectum, and lower abdomen; paittika piles are delicate, mobile, pale, and resemble a parrots tongue; they are moist and spindle shaped and are accompanied by blood in stools, burning sensation, thirst, and general signs of pallor; kaphaja piles are pale, fixed, broad-based, yellowish white, and resemble the kernel of a panasa fruit, with copious mucus discharge and much itching; raktaja piles look like the sprouts of a banyan tree and bleed profusely, when pressed by hard stools. When three or two doṣas are mixed, the clinical features will also be mixed.

Though, hereditary piles are caused by vitiation of sperm and ovum and have various general findings such as venous engorgement elsewhere in the body, feeble voice, irritability, and lethargy; the treatment of hereditary piles follows the same methods as for other types of piles.[18]

"Piles" may appear elsewhere in the body such as genitalia, umbilical region, and lips, but we shall not be dealing with their treatment.

Management of piles: Medical treatment including caustics, cautery, and surgery are employed in the management of piles on the basis of the clinical features of the disease. In general, medical treatment is advised, when the symptoms are minimal, piles are hardly visible and perturbation of doṣas is insignificant; caustics are used when pile masses are soft, deeply located and projecting, and covers a wide area; thermal cautery is advised when the piles are rough, firm, and solid; lastly, surgery is preferred when the projecting pile masses have a narrow peduncle and have a moist surface.[19]

Caustics:[20] Patients should undergo lubricant therapy and fomentation and should have been taking a liquid and bland diet for a few days prior to the procedure. On the prefixed day in good weather, he should be placed on a flat and hard wooden bed with the anus facing the sun to gain maximum visibility. He should be supine with the upper part of his body resting on the lap of an attendant. His waist should be elevated by a roll of cloth, neck, and legs fixed firmly by a strap and the positions firmly maintained by strong attendants. After lubricating the anus, the proctoscope is introduced into the rectum, while the patient strains and the pile masses come into view. The pile masses should be pressed and dried by a cotton swab held on a probe (śalāka). Then, the caustic should be applied on a pile mass for a hundred mātras (mātra is the time taken to pronounce a short vowel). It may be applied again until the piles assume a bluish, black colour of jambū fruit and shrinks. The caustic is then washed away by gruel, yoghurt, and buttermilk. The pile mass is then daubed with ghee and madhuka. The patient should sit in a warm water bath for a while and sent back to his room for rest. If there is more than one pile mass, caustic should be applied to one at a time at weekly intervals.

Vātika and kaphaja pile should be treated by caustics and cautery; raktaja and pittaja types should be managed by mild caustics only. Depending on the visual characteristics of the piles seen through the speculum, patient's strength and doṣa status, the pile mass may be cauterized or excised through the speculum.

SS discusses in detail the signs of under, over, and optimum use of caustics, and complications of using caustic. There is also an excellent description of the rectal speculum with two holes – in - one for visualization and the other for caustics application. The drugs and medical pastes used for oral and local use in the medical treatment of piles and doṣa perturbation in piles and a bhallātaka regime in treatment are also described in great detail.[21]

Suśruta cautioned that caustics, cautery, and piles excision in the rectum through a speculum should be used with utmost care. Incorrect use could cause serious complications such as impotence, abdominal distention, constipation or diarrhoea, and even death.

The decline of Suśruta's surgical legacy

The moving words of Kāśirāja Divodāsa - Suśruta's teacher - in his tribute to surgery bear testimony to the glory that was "śalya" in ancient India. Suśruta blazed a trail by setting up a "Dhanvantari school" for surgery in Banaras and composing an authoritative text in Āyurveda with a surgical orientation, which continues to be admired and taught even after the passage of 25 centuries. For describing innovative operations such as the plastic reconstruction of a deformed nose, for developing a whole series of 120 instruments for varied surgical procedures, for setting up a programme in experimental surgery for the training of surgeons and above all, for demonstrating in his life that surgery is more than operations, Suśruta will always shine as an inspirational figure in India's scientific firmament.

In Buddha's life, we come across another stellar figure - Jīvaka who is largely forgotten in India, but was a surgeon extraordinary and the physician of Lord Buddha and King Bimbisara. Buddhist literature has many interesting anecdotes about his humble origin as an orphan, his training as a brilliant physician under Ātreya in Takṣaśilā and triumphant return to Rajagir as a successful surgeon and royal physician. Nothing written by him has survived, but there are vivid accounts of his trephining the skull of a very sick merchant, removing two worms and giving dramatic relief to him. He successfully operated on King Bimbisara for anal fistula as well. In Buddhist India, great universities such as Takṣaśilā - the alma mater of Jīvaka - and Nalanda flourished and drew students from all over North India and neighbouring countries. Apart from Buddhist philosophy, the main subject taught in the universities was Āyurveda, which was an inseparable and highly respected part of the curriculum. Suśruta and Jīvaka were revered as Ācaryas and an admiring Hieun Tsang was saddened to observe the residence of Jīvaka in ruins next to the hall, also in ruins, which he had built for Lord Buddha to give his sermons.

However, the palmy days of surgery developed atrophic changes of unknown origin towards the beginning of the current era. The manifestations of atrophy are undeniable. The surgical procedures described by Suśruta including the treatment of fractures gradually faded from the mainstream of Āyurveda and Vaidyas no longer performed them; dissection of cadavers to learn human anatomy - even though practiced in rotting bodies -became a distant memory, and references to surgery became minimal in Ayurvedic texts. Whereas, Ayurvedic texts such as those of Sāraṅgadhara, Mādhava, and Bhāva Miśra and Nighaṇṭus continued to appear during the long phase of stagnation of Āyurveda after Vāgbhaṭa, the springs of surgical texts simply ran dry. It was as if the sun had set on Suśruta's surgical legacy too soon.

A closer look at the "darkness at noon," which cast its shadow on surgery reveals a disturbing trend of social and cultural regression. Incredible as it may seem, we find that surgical procedures such as plastic reconstruction of the nose, couching for cataract, and reduction of fractures, which were pioneered by Suśruta had not only disappeared from the mainstream of Āyurveda, but had passed on to the hands of illiterate, traditional practitioners who belonged to "lower castes" and were denied education and social mobility. Thanks to this condemnable exercise in social engineering, all those who used their hands to make a living, to make things of beauty and utility for the society, and who had been respected all along found themselves downgraded as lower castes. Indeed, surgeons were ineligible to attend auspicious ceremonies! The sophisticated operations such as the plastic repair of the nose and the making of the famous wootz steel by India's craftsmen reincarnated among the "lower castes," who had no formal education and had learnt their skills from their father or guardian in their home. While Indians apparently kept no records of these sombre developments, they were carefully observed and recorded by British observers in the 18th century.

A "coomar caste" man doing a plastic repair of the nose under a tree in Pune, a Mohammedan doing a couching for cataract in a public place in Coimbatore, an illiterate worker building a furnace and refinery in his backyard in Madhya Pradesh and making steel of high quality, a travelling band from UP visiting Bengal every year to practice "Tikka" (variolation) to prevent small pox, and other examples illustrate the colossal injustice done by Indians against themselves, which could only lead the society to slavery and ruin. British observers who were quite competent and had watched the Indians at work during the plastic operation and making steel did ask them many questions about their methods, why they were being done in a particular way, why not in some other way, and so on, as they were impressed by the skill and high quality of the work being done. But, the replies to all questions were similar "I do not know"; this is what my father taught me and this is the best way to do this job.*

(The reports of British observers on several of these examples are given in the complete works of Dharampal Vol. 1 Indian Science and Technology in the Eighteenth century. Other Indian Press, Goa 2000.)*

The "surgeons," weavers, metal craftsmen, artisans, and others who did the work could not answer any questions on "why" with reference to what they were doing. About this shocking observation, P C Ray made these scathing remarks:

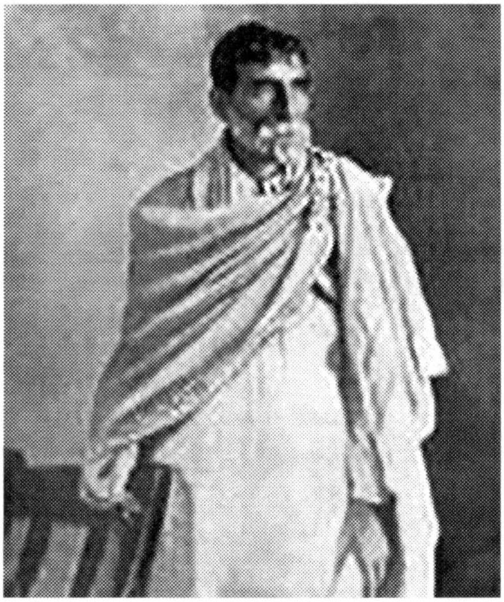

Figure 15: P C Ray

> According to Suśruta, 'the dissection of dead bodies is a sine qua non to the student of surgery, and this high authority lays particular stress on knowledge gained from experiments and observations.
>
> But Manu would have none of it. The very touch of a corpse, according to Manu, is enough to bring contamination to the sacred person of a Brāhmana. Thus, we find that shortly after the time of Vāgbhaṭa, the handling of lancet was discouraged, and anatomy and surgery fell into disuse and became, to all intents and purposes, lost sciences to the Hindus. It was considered equally undignified to sweat away at the forge like a Cyclops. Hence, the cultivation of Kalās by the more refined classes of the society, of which we get a vivid picture in the ancient Sanskrit literature, has survived only in traditions since a very long time past.
>
> The arts thus being relegated to the lower castes, and the professions made hereditary, a certain degree of deftness in manipulation was no doubt secured, but this was at a terrible cost. The intellectual portion of the community being thus withdrawn from active participation in arts, the how and why of phenomena – the coordination of cause and effect

– were lost sight of. The spirit of enquiry gradually died out among a nation, naturally prone to speculation and metaphysical subtleties, and India for once bade adieu to experimental and inductive sciences. Her soil was made morally unfit for the birth of a Boyle, a Descartes, or a Newton, and her very name was all but expunged from the map of the scientific world for a time.'[22]

Under these circumstances, India's rout in the East-West encounter of the 18th century was a foregone conclusion. The lesson for us from this suicidal folly is never to dissociate hand from the head or to regard craftsmanship as inferior to "brain work" lest we should forever be condemned to the death of innovation and intellectual barrenness.

References:

1. *CS* Nidāna 15: 8 – 10
2. *SS* Cikitsā 3: 4 – 5
3. *SS* Cikitsā 3: 17 – 21
4. *SS* Cikitsā 3: 23 – 27
5. *SS* Nidāna 15: 11 – 15
6. *SS* Cikitsā 3: 6 – 14
7. *SS* Cikitsā 3: 55 – 68
8. *SS* Sūtra 16: 27 – 31
9. *SS* Sūtra 26: 4 – 6
10. *SS* Sūtra 26: 9 – 13
11. *SS* Sūtra 26: 15 – 21
12. *SS* Sūtra 27: 3 – 5
13. *SS* Sūtra 27: 6 – 12
14. *SS* Sūtra 27: 14
15. *SS* Sūtra 27: 19 – 24
16. *SS* Nidāna 2: 4
17. *SS* Nidāna 2: 7
18. *SS* Nidāna 2: 10 – 16
19. *SS* Cikitsā 6: 3
20. *SS* Cikitsā 6: 15
21. *SS* Cikitsā 6: 12 – 18
22. P C Ray. *A History of Hindu Chemistry*. Shaibya Prakashan Bibhag 1902. First Ed. Vol 1 Pages 195 – 96.

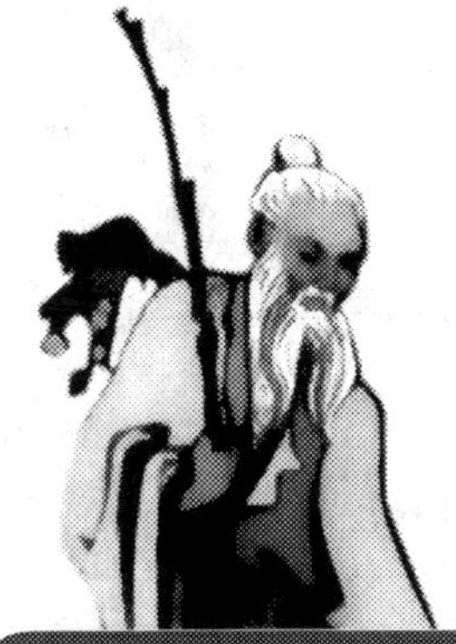

CHAPTER 14

Rejuvenation (Rasāyana) and Enhancement of Sexual Potency (Vājīkaraṇa)

Rejuvenation and Vājīkaraṇa are two branches of Āyurveda, which claimed serious attention from Caraka, Suśruta, and Vāgbhaṭa. This would be a surprise to many who shared a long held, but thoroughly mistaken, view that Indians are fatalistic and pessimistic, preferring a life of renunciation and aspiration for a life hereafter. As we noted, Caraka explicitly declared in the beginning of his Saṃhitā, that the first two urges in life are longevity and a life in comfort. After-life came third but it was, according to him, enmeshed in doubt. His attitude to life was cheerful, if not roseate, and neither he, nor Suśruta, nor Vāgbhaṭa forbade any kind of enjoyment provided it did not violate good conduct. Eating was not only to satisfy a biological urge, but also to be enjoyed; sexual activity was not only for procreation, but also for enjoyment which was a part of it. It was therefore natural that Āyurveda would seek to eliminate the infirmities of ageing, which make life miserable in the final years. Āyurveda recognized that ageing and death are biological events, which are not preventable but it also urged, based on experience, that many of the infirmities of senses, organs and parts of the body could be prevented and their adverse effects mitigated by good conduct and medical measures.

Rejuvenation (Rasāyana)

Medicaments (bheṣaja) are of two kinds; those which augment the strength and resistance of the healthy, and others which counter diseases. In the category of medicaments or drugs which promote strength, there are two groups; those which enhance the strength, resistance to disease, and sense of well-being, and others which promote sexual potency and fecundity. This categorization is not absolute because there may be overlaps in the functions of drugs, which promote good health and those which combat diseases.[1] The promotive group increases longevity, memory, intellect, complexion, voice, physical strength, and youthful ageing and are called rasāyana, a subgroup of this is designated Vājīkaraṇa as it enhances sexual potency like that of a horse and fecundity, which ensures the survival of one's lineage and reputation.

Rasāyana in ageing: Mechanism of action

Rasāyana or rejuvenative therapy is specifically recommended to ward off age-related infirmities and promote youthful ageing. Ageing is not a disease, but a normal biological process inherent in all dhātus. The dhātus, which constitute the body are constantly depleting as the etymology of "śārīra" suggests. Dhātus include "rasa," which is the essence of āhārarasa derived from the digestion of what one eats and drinks. The function of "rasāyana" is to convey "rasa" to the destination or dhātus; it would also ease the passage of rasa to the dhātus. As age advances, rasa derived from food and drinks may decrease due to poor appetite and intake of food, weak digestion of food in the stomach, narrowing of channels (srotas) transporting substances to the dhātus all over the body, and slowing down of digestive fires in the dhātus. Rasāyana acts at all these levels, from the gross to the subtle. In Āyurveda, "sukha" is synonymous with good health and wellness. Etymologically "kham" means channels (srotas) and "suṣṭu" signifies "appropriateness." A state of "sukha" would therefore imply the appropriate state or patency of channels, which is precisely what rasāyana aims to achieve. Rasāyana improves appetite, digestion in the stomach, transport of rasa resulting from āhārarasa to the dhātus, and the utilization of the rasa by agnis (fires) in the dhātus as the agnis tend to slow down in the dhātus during ageing.

It is however, necessary to fulfill prescribed requirements for the rasāyana procedure to succeed. It should start for an individual in mid-forties, when the degenerative changes in the dhātus would not have progressed to a stage, when they have become irreversible. In a subject past 60 or 70, the decrease in the level of agnis in the stomach and dhātus and the narrowing of body channels would impede the functioning of rasāyana and the result of treatment would be limited. Furthermore, a virtuous code of conduct is obligatory and binding on an individual in order to gain the full benefit of rasāyana therapy. Vāgbhaṭa defined "truthfulness, freedom from anger, habit of introspection, spiritual orientation of mind, tranquility, and observance of virtuous conduct" as indispensable for the effective practice of Rasāyana.[2] Rasāyana therapy, which violates the code and reduces it to the mere intake of formulations is unlikely to give benefits for an individual.

Rasāyana procedure: Rasāyana procedure is carried out by two different methods. The indoor method (kuṭipraveśika) is rigorous, expensive, and more effective; but the eligibility is restricted to those who are healthy, physically fit, intelligent, self-controlled, affluent, and are free from disease. Kuṭipraveśika is superior, but it is very difficult.[3] Individuals, who fall short of the tough requirements should opt for the easier and more relaxed method of vātātapika, which is practiced outdoors and is compatible with one's occupation and a common man's life style.

Kuṭipraveśika requires a specially built residential facility or hut in a quiet location, free from wind and dust, facing the east or the north, and painted in white. In the circular space within, there should be three concentric walls with a door on each, which are not aligned. The entry from one circular corridor to the next would be through the doors only and the room in the center should be spacious enough for the subject to live for several days and for the physician to attend to him. In this special hut, one would be isolated, and sheltered from sun, smoke, wind, company of women and men except for the attending physician and attendant from time to time. The subject should enter the hut on an auspicious day and moment and undergo purification by bath and pañcakarma procedure. He should pay homage to the gods, physician and Brāhmaṇas, chant propitiatory hymns, entertain only good thoughts, and speak only wholesome words. No visitors should be permitted except the physician and attendant, who serve him food and rasāyanas at prefixed timings.

Following the purificatory procedure of pañcakarma, a dietary regime consisting mainly of milk or gruel should be instituted depending on the subjects' constitution, season, and response to the regime for a few days. This would be followed by one meal a day and two or three dozes of rasāyanas, which are based on numerous classical formulae described by Caraka, Suśruta, and Vāgbhaṭa. They are based on traditional drugs such as āmalakī, harītakī, śalaparṇī, pippalī, śankapuṣpī, viḍaṅga, nāgabala, and others and have well-known names such as aindra rasāyana, āmalakī rasāyana, brāhmi rasāyana, and nārasimha rasāyana. The physician would decide on the choice of a rasāyana, its dosage, and frequency of administration, keeping in mind the subject's tolerance to the dietary regimen and rasāyana in the new environment. If he gets indigestion, the regimen should be revised. The treatment would continue from 7 to 28 days, when the rasāyana would have reached and impinged on all the dhātus of the subject. If the protocol is breached, such as the hut is improperly designed, purificatory procedure is not properly done, the dietary regimen is incorrect, a wrong rasāyana, or wrong dosage of the appropriate rasāyana is given, the kuṭipraveśika method may fail or might even produce adverse reactions. It would appear that this method was used in practice only by saints, who wished to fortify themselves for a harsh life of penance or by kings and affluent persons in ancient India.

In 20th century, kuṭipraveśika was famously practiced by Pandit Madan Mohan Malaviya in the Banaras University. The procedure was then known as kāyakalpa. Malaviyaji was 77 years old, when he decided to undergo kāyakalpa under the direction of Tapsi Baba who was a saintly person and an expert in the procedure against the advice of the Professor of Āyurveda in the University. For the initial ten days, he showed improvement by gain in weight, improvement in memory, and vision and a general sense of well-being. However, he experienced sleeplessness and other disturbances and the procedure was terminated prematurely instead of continuing for 40 days as planned originally. The trial was therefore inconclusive.[4]

The outdoor method of rasāyana termed vātātapika, as the name implies, exposes the subject to wind and sun and is more suitable for individuals who work for a living. This method is not rigorous and permits the individual to take one main meal a day and consume the rasāyana formulation prescribed by the physician for 30 days. Lapses in the procedure do not involve complications. Vāgbhaṭa's list of formulations numbered 30 and other Ācāryas prescribed many more. But, all authorities agreed that this method too would be futile in the absence of virtuous conduct by the subject. Two examples of the rasāyana formulations are given in Table 1:

Table 1: Rasāyana Formulations-Two examples

Sl No	Formulations	Actions	Comments
1.	Fruits of āmalaka, harītaki, bibhītaka (āmalakī rasāyana)	Regaining youth, freedom from illness, strength, intellectual ability	Different combinations of the three fruits wrapped in palāśa bark; covered with mud and baked. It is then, powdered and taken with curd, ghee, etc., as per directions.
2.	Red hot iron leaves dipped in decoction of iṅgudi, triphala, palāśa, and āmalakī juice (lauhādi rasāyana)	Promotes strength, scholarship, eloquence	Processed as per detailed protocol and powdered. Mixed with honey and ghee and preserved for a year. Gold and silver added in some protocols.

Rasāyanas: Fanciful claims

It is interesting that Ayurvedic texts make exaggerated claims on the effects of Rasāyana and Vājīkaraṇa. It is common to read about significant improvement in physical activity, freedom from ailments, enhancement in cognitive and sensory functions, and sexual vigour following the proper use of rasāyanas. However, it is also common to read about subjects being rewarded by living for many centuries free from disease (Caraka and Suśruta), making a man invisible (Caraka), vision of goddess Sri (Caraka), maintaining erection all night for sexual activity (Caraka), a man of eighty getting erectile power of a young man (Suśruta), and so on. These claims stand in sharp contrast to the descriptions of treating diseases and their prognosis in terms of curability, curability with difficulty, and incurability in ancient texts. In the former, the classics seem to reflect popular beliefs uncritically, whereas, the latter describe the practice of medicine as it then was with objectivity and realism. Alternately, an imaginative and unscrupulous physician could have inserted the fanciful descriptions in ancient classics of masters.

Enhancement of sexual potency and fecundity (Vājīkaraṇa)

Vājīkaraṇa is a branch of Āyurveda, which deals with measures to enhance sexual potency and fecundity. It largely consists of a number of formulations, many belonging to animal products, which are used in treating erectile dysfunction. This was a subject of importance as it received serious attention from Caraka, Suśruta, and Vāgbhaṭa. Caraka held the view that healthy and self-confident men should regularly take vṛṣya drugs (drugs which enhance erectile function), which not only enhance sexual potency but also pleasure, wealth, and fame besides giving male offspring. After giving an eloquent description of a beautiful woman who captures one's heart as the best vṛṣya drug, Caraka heaped praise on a man who produces numerous progeny and ridiculed one who is unable to produce offspring. The conclusion was obvious because vṛṣya drugs held the key for enhancing both sexual potency and fecundity.[5] Thereafter, he proceeded to describe a long list of drugs, their composition and preparation, and the promised results. Suśruta is more systematic in dealing with Vājīkaraṇa. While, vṛṣya drugs enable a healthy adult to perform sexual intercourse on any day in any season, they are necessary to treat the elderly, sexually insatiable, impotent, polygamous, and those deficient in semen. However, he concurred with Caraka that the best among vṛṣya drugs is a beautiful woman.[6]

Suśruta classified impotence (klaibya) into six types as follows:[7]

- Mind is suddenly overpowered by improper or frightful thoughts during foreplay or sexual intercourse, causing immediate flaccidity and impotence.
- Ingestion of large quantities of pungent/sour/salty food items.
- Those in the habit of taking vṛṣya drugs do intercourse without taking them.
- Diseases or injury to the penis.
- No erection from adolescence – congenital type.

- Those practicing brahmacarya for many years may develop hardening of semen and impotence. Except the congenital type and that due to disease or injury to the penis, all other types are amenable to treatment by vṛṣya drugs.[8]

A few examples of the formulations recommended are given below:[9]

Table 2: Examples-Formulations

Formulations	Method of preparations	Comments
Powdered tila, māṣa, vidari	Mixed with pauṇḍraka, sugar cane juice, ground with saindhava, and animal fat, and cooked in ghee	Gains erectile power to satisfy a hundred women
Goat's testicles	Cooked in ghee, extracted with milk, pippalī, and salt added	Same as above
Black gram	Mixed with honey and ghee: Followed by milk drink	Strong sexual stimulant

A new look at Rasāyana

Vāgbhaṭa's statement on Ayurvedic practices, "These are to be done not only because they are recorded in scriptural texts, but also because they show demonstrable results. They can be administered without any debate as if they are sacred mantras"[10] is significant because "demonstrable results" were insisted upon for a procedure to be accepted in his time. Faith alone was no longer sufficient, which had been anticipated by Caraka more than a 1000 year before Vāgbhaṭa. He had proclaimed the shift of Ayurvedic practice from a faith-based (daivavyapāśraya) to a reason-based (yuktivyapāśraya) platform. Fifteen centuries after Vāgbhaṭa, his successors may be forgiven for seeking "demonstrable results" of a different kind in the present century, which resounds with clarion calls for "evidence-based medicine" and even "evidence-based Āyurveda". As far as rasāyanas are concerned, a question would arise, "Do the ancient texts give any clues, which would lend themselves to a study of the mechanism of action of rasāyana with the tools of current science?" This question was, in fact, taken up for a study by Professor Subba Rao and colleagues in the JNTU, Hyderabad in 2012 as they had considerable experience in accurately measuring the breakup of DNA in the brain cells of rats and felt, after discussions with biological scientists and Vaidyas of Arya Vaidya Śala, Kottakkal, that āmalakī rasāyana could be easily administered to the rats and its effect, if any, on the brain cells measured at intervals of three, nine, and fifteen months as they had been doing quite successfully for other experiments for many years.

Rats have a life span of two years and their DNA in brain cells begins to show breakages by the age of three months, which keep on increasing to very high levels by 15 months. Breakages in DNA mean decline in function of the cells, which would signify the slow but certain deterioration of brain function until the animals are almost "brain dead" before the end of their life span. When the rats were fed their usual ration with a supplement of āmalakī rasāyana made in Arya Vaidya Śala, as per the formula of Vāgbhaṭa, the scientists in Hyderabad observed that the DNA breaks were significantly less at three months compared to the rats not taking the rasāyana; the difference became progressively greater at nine months and maximum at 15 months. In other words, rasāyana gave stability to the DNA of brain cells as the rats were getting older.[11] This is after all one of the benefits of rasāyanas, which protect and enhance brain function. This is evidence to convince the tough scientific judges of the 21st century, but that was not all.

Professor Lakhotia and colleagues in the Banaras Hindu University have been doing research in genetics for years with fruit flies – *Drosophila melanogaster* - as their model. These flies are the international favourites of geneticists because their life span is only 30 days and the events in an entire life time can be observed in one month. It is true that fruit flies are vastly different from humans, but there is much that they share with humans in genetic structure and biological response to various stresses in life. Furthermore, by transferring the genes responsible for certain human diseases to the fruit fly, the disease features have been reproduced faithfully in the humble fly, which is "genetically engineered." Professor Lakhotia and colleagues enriched the diet of the flies with āmalakī rasāyana and found that their life span, fecundity in terms of eggs laid, tolerance of heat, tolerance of starvation, and other biological markers were greatly improved in the flies consuming the rasāyana-enriched diet compared to the control flies, who had only their usual ration without rasāyana.[12] They reconfirmed these results by several subsequent studies, which were published.

Another group of scientists led by Professor C C Kartha at the Rajiv Gandhi Centre for Biotechnology, Trivandrum have studied the effect of āmalakī rasāyana on the thickening of heart muscle wall in response to high blood pressure and their results suggest that the rasāyana has protective effect on the heart muscle. These studies on three different models on the rat brain, fruit fly, and rat heart strongly suggest that the rasāyana does have a protective/promotive effect on multiple biological systems. These experiments are merely a beginning because the effect of many other rasāyanas on different biological models would reveal a great deal more about how the rasāyanas bring about the observed effects. As we search more – the research in science is unending – we would learn more about ageing, how the rasāyana works and how we may, as successors of our great physician – scientists of yore, hope to develop even better rasāyanas to mitigate human suffering.

References:

1. *CS Cikitsā* 1: 4–12
2. *Vāgbhaṭa AH Uttara* 39:179
3. *CS Cikitsā* 1: 27–29
4. *Paramanand: Mahamana Madan Mohan Malaviya*. BHU. 1985, Vol. II: Pages 992–1004.
5. *CS Cikitsā* II: 1.3–23
6. *SS Cikitsā* 26: 3–8
7. *SS Cikitsā* 26: 9–15
8. *SS Cikitsā* 26: 9–15
9. *SS Cikitsā* 26: 16–19
10. *Vāgbhaṭa AH Uttara* 40: 81
11. Studies on the molecular correlates of genomic stability in rat brain cells following Āmalakīrasayana therapy. Umakanta Swain, Kiran Kumar Sindhu, Ushasri Boda, Suresh Pothani, Nappan V Giridharan, Manchala Raghunath, and Kalluri Subba Rao. *Mechanisms of Ageing and Development*, April 133(4):112-117, (2012).
12. *In Vivo Effects of Traditional Ayurvedic Formulations in Drosophila Melanogaster Model Relate with Therapeutic Applications*. Vibha Dwivedi, E M Anandan, Rajesh S Mony, T S Muraleedharan, M S Valiathan, Mousumi Mutsuddi, and Subhash C Lakhotia. PLoS ONE, 7(5), e37113, (2012).

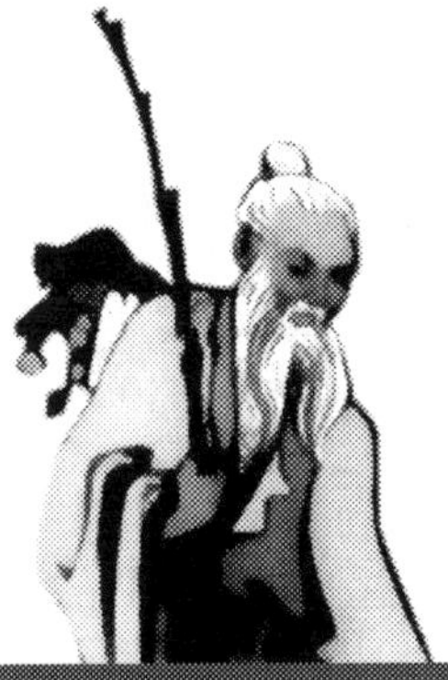

CHAPTER 15

Training of a Physician

Early education: Gurukula

In ancient India, the education of pupils took place primarily in the Gurukula, where they lived in the teacher's house. They learnt reading, writing, arithmetic (gaṇita), Vedic literature, smṛitis, purāṇas, arthaśāstra, daṇḍanīti (politics), anvīkṣikī (physical sciences), and crafts. Though writing was known and practiced, learning by rote was probably more popular. The role of the teacher was exalted far above that of written texts in the Gurukulas. Over several years, the students would acquire sufficient knowledge and develop interests of their own to become a physician, philosopher, expert in warfare, or administrator, which would call for training at another level. The life in the Gurukula not only gave the pupil the basic knowledge required to pursue specialized studies in subjects like medicine, but also greatly influenced his life in its totality. The pupil left the home of his parents at a tender age to live in the home of his Guru for several years, when the very meaning of his life would change for him. Unless he had done credit to himself in the Gurukula, he could not hope to enter for training as a physician as the standards set by Caraka for admission, as we shall see, were very high.

Normally, the teacher in the Gurukula would not charge any fees from pupils, who lived in the house and offered services for the household such as fetching fire wood, cooking, running errands, and so on. The teacher maintained strict discipline and pupils had to work hard. Physical fitness was an essential requirement for admission to a Gurukula as one finds references to studious pupils working day and night and, when they ran out of oil for a lamp, burning cow dung to read in its light in a solitary corner. Indifferent or lazy students would drop out and others who violated discipline would be dismissed. Famous teachers, who would attract pupils from hundreds of miles away, were venerated as "yaujanaśatika." Neither teachers, who charged fees nor pupils who paid for education were highly regarded. At the conclusion of training in a Gurukula, the pupil was expected to give a gift (Dakṣiṇā) according to his capacity such as field, gold, cow, horse, umbrella, or shoes. An old verse summed up the process of learning thus: "The pupil learns a quarter from the teacher; a quarter from his own intellectual effort; a quarter from his fellow students; and the last quarter from what life teaches him."

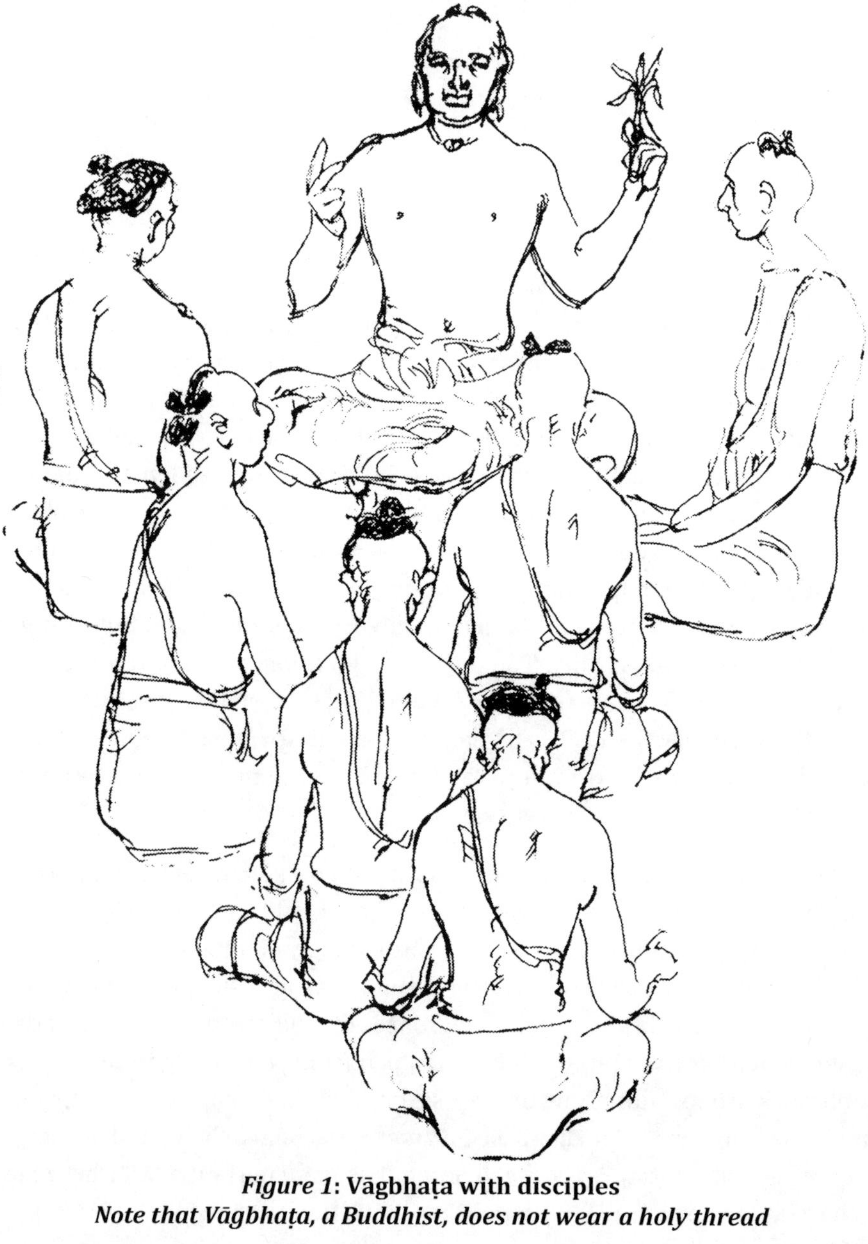

***Figure 1*: Vāgbhaṭa with disciples**
Note that Vāgbhaṭa, a Buddhist, does not wear a holy thread

Aśrama (Hermitage)

Caraka Saṃhitā (CS), redacted from Agniveśatantra written many centuries earlier, refers to the origin of the Agniveśa text. Ācārya Punarvasu Ātreya had six disciples in his Āśrama – Agniveśa, Bhela, Jatukarṇa, Parāśāra, Hārīta, and Kṣārapāṇi, on whom he had bestowed his knowledge of Āyurveda out of friendliness (maitrīpara). He taught them all subjects in equal measure without differentiation. Each disciple composed a book based on his understanding of what had been taught and presented it before an assembly of sages presided over by Ātreya. The assembly unanimously praised all the compositions, but their special acclamation was lavished on Agniveśa in so far as they proclaimed that the goddesses of intelligence (buddhi), success (siddhi), memory (smṛti), intellect (medhā), firmness (dhṛti), fame (kīrti), patience (kṣamā), and kindness (dayā) had unitedly blessed the text of Agniveśa.[1] This description reveals that Ātreya's āśrama admitted a limited number of students; they were among the brightest to be chosen for admission from among the alumni of Gurukulas. The duration of training and erudite atmosphere in the āśrama were such that it was an intellectual power house, which transformed bright seekers of medicine into physician – scholars in the mould of Agniveśa.

A student seeking to be a physician: Given his strong credentials in liberal education in the Gurukula and scholarly effort on his own, a student should select an authoritative treatise in Āyurveda as the basic text for study. It should have high seriousness and repute; it should be used by wise men and scholars, it should be full of ideas, lucid, intelligible even to the dull, and free from the error of repetition. It should have a sage's lineage, a logical and well prepared introduction and discussions on traditional ideas leading to the understanding of their essence, and internal consistency. It should give examples to illustrate definitions, exclude difficult words and serve like the sun in throwing light on entire subjects and eliminating the darkness of ignorance.

The seeker should also consider the teacher and ascertain his qualities: Does he have a good understanding of the subject? Does he have practical experience? Is he friendly and clean? Does he have necessary equipment for instruction? Is he even tempered? Does he know human nature? Is he free from envy and anger? Is he patient and fatherly to the students? These qualities of the teacher will soon get instilled in the student. He should approach the teacher and salute him with the combined reverence shown to fire god, king, father, and mother. Through his pleasure, the student should acquire knowledge of the entire treatise and strive constantly to strengthen his understanding, improve his expression, and ability to speak.[2]

Method of study: There are three methods, which are - study on one's own (adhyayana), discourse by the teacher (adhyāpana), and discussion (sambhāṣā). As soon as the student wakes up before dawn, he should perform morning ablutions and offer prayers to gods, sages, cow, brāhmaṇa, teachers, and elders and sit down comfortably in a quiet place. He should recite the verse or aphorisms learnt in a clear voice repeatedly and try to understand them in depth. He should continue this effort during mid-day, afternoon, and night.

To teach, the teacher should make sure that the student is eligible to be taught. This would oblige him to enquire: Does he have a calm and noble nature? Does he have good features, eyes, and a sharp nasal bridge? Is his tongue thin, red, and clean? Does he have any deformity of teeth or lips and does he have a nasal voice? Is he vain? Does he have self-restraint, power of reasoning, intelligence, and good memory? Is he broadminded and from a family of physicians? Is he truthful? Are his senses in order? Is he free from anger, greed, and bad habits? Is he sincere, skillful, modest, and keen in study? Is he compassionate to all creatures? If the teacher is satisfied after these enquiries, he should choose an auspicious day in the bright fortnight during the northern course of the sun and favourable astral combination for initiation and say to the student, "You come to me after tonsuring your head, fasting overnight and bath, wearing ochre cloth, and a sacred thread. You should bring with you - firewood, fire, ghee, paste, water jars, garland, rope, lamp, vessels of gold and silver, precious stones, milk, sticks to mark the auspicious platform, darbhā grass, fried paddy, mustard seeds, barley grains, white flowers, and sattvic food."[3]

The third method of study – Sambhāṣā – is taken up after the disciple's initiation is over.

Initiation Ceremony: The platform for the ceremony should be four cubits on even ground, sloping towards the east or the north. The platform should be plastered with cow dung, covered with darbhā grass, and provided with the previously listed articles and bounded by sticks. A fire should be lit with fuel sticks of palāśa, iṅgudī, udumbara, and madhuka and the teacher should offer oblations as prescribed while invoking mantras dedicated to Brahma, Agni, Dhanvantari, Prajāpati, Aśvins, Indra, and sages. The chants should end with "svāha" thrice. The disciple should repeat the chants after the teacher. The assembled brāhmaṇas should chant "svasti" and the disciple should pay homage to the physicians in the assembly.[4] (Figure 2)

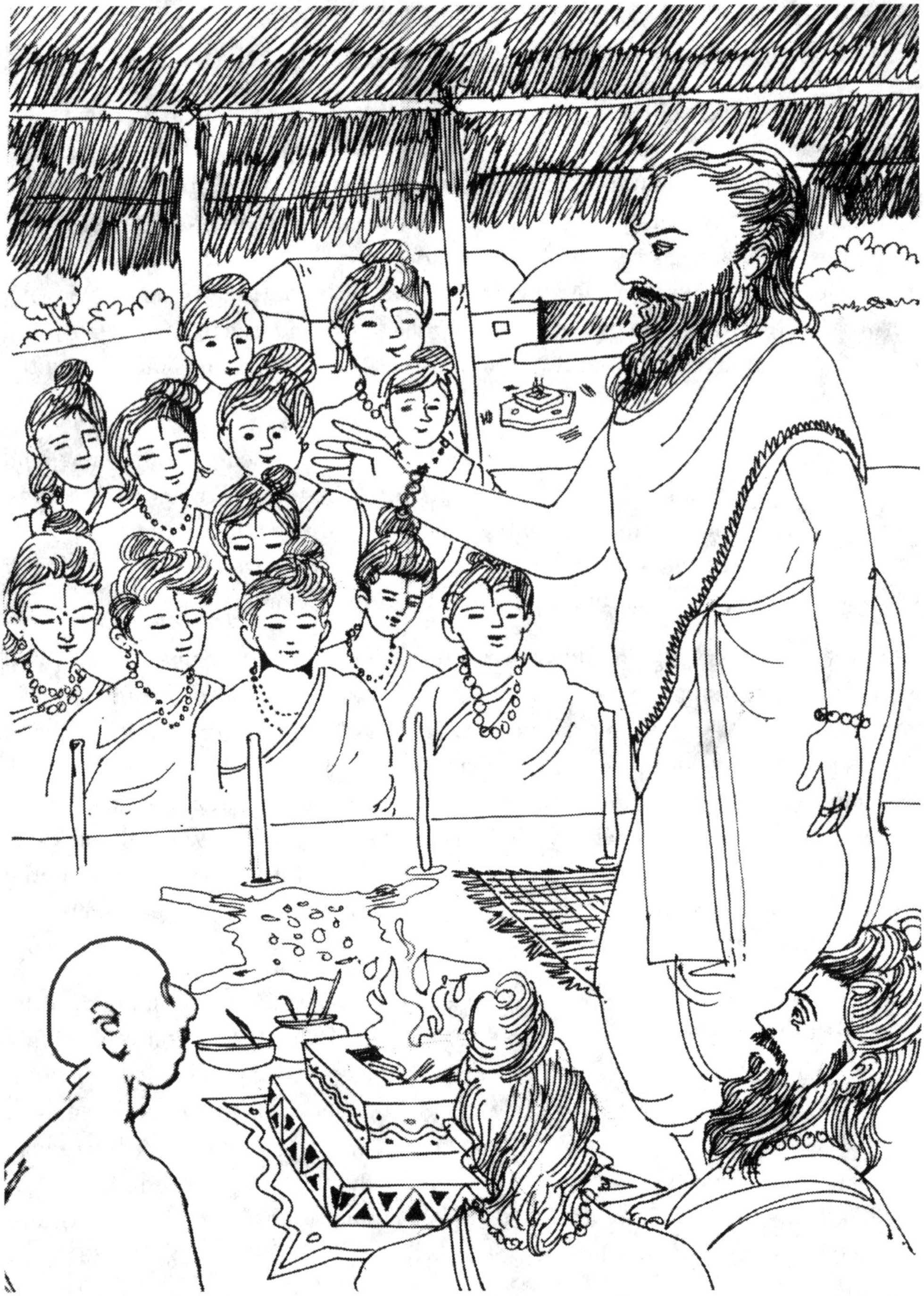

Figure 2: Ācārya administering the oath on initiation, to a medical trainee before the sacrificial fire as witness and learned assembly.

Disciple's oath on initiation: In the open assembly with the sacrificial fire as witness, the teacher should command the disciple as follows:

"You shall observe celibacy, speak the truth, abstain from meat and eat only intellect-promoting (medhyasevi) food; you should carry no weapons; you should never disobey my commands except when you face the king's wrath, danger to your life, or some other calamity. You should always be subject to me, submissive to me, and follow the path charted by me; you should live with me as my son, servant, and dependent and regard me as your master; you should move about with my permission, with presence of mind, humility, vigilance, and free from arrogance and jealousy. You should move about in the first place to collect things for me and the household.

When you join the ranks of physicians and aspire for success, wealth, fame, and a happy afterlife, you should always keep in mind the welfare of all living beings, cows, and brāhmaṇas in the forefront; you should spare no effort to save the health of patients and never entertain low thoughts about them even at the cost of your life; you should not even dream of approaching others' women or property.

Your dress and bearing should be simple, you should shun drinking, sins, and association with sinners; your words should be gentle, pure, proper, joyous, appreciative, truthful, and measured; you should always be mindful of place and time, keep memory sharp, and make ceaseless effort to acquire knowledge, skill, and improve the quality of equipment; you should refuse to treat persons hostile to the king or who are disliked by the king or by noble persons, who are incurably diseased and those who are wicked; you should also refuse to treat women in the absence of their husbands or guardians, nor should you accept meat offered by women without the permission of their husbands or guardians.

While entering a house, you should be accompanied by a person known to the family; you should be decently dressed, head bowed, quiet, thoughtful, and moving gracefully; you should not talk or use your sense organs during the visit except with reference to the patient, his illness and well-being. The information received from within the house should never be revealed outside; even if you know the patient's life span is short, you should not disclose it lest it should cause agony to the patient and his relatives. Even if you are learned, you should not brag because people are irritated by bragging even from experts.

Āyurveda has no end and one must always engage in its study diligently. It is worthwhile to learn agreeable conduct without jealousy even from enemies because the whole world is a teacher for the wise. One should therefore give due consideration to advice which is appreciative, promoting fame, life span, strength, and good will among people.

You should conduct yourself with respect towards gods, fire, brāhmaṇas, teacher, elders, and noble ones; then the fire with all the perfumes, eatables, gems, and grains will grant you prosperity otherwise they will curse you." When the teacher concludes thus, the disciple should say "yes". If the disciple obeys the teacher, he should be taught, otherwise not.[5]

Discussion (Sambhāṣā):[6] Caraka had mentioned three methods of study namely, studying on one's own, discourse by the teacher, and discussion. Before taking up the subject of discussion, he stopped to consider the initiation of disciples into the study of Āyurveda and the procedures associated with it. The probable reason for this detour is that discussion plays an even greater role in a physician's career than in a disciple's life. After all, the training of a physician is a lifelong process. Caraka urged that a physician should hold discussions with physicians because they advance the frontiers of knowledge, add to skills, make one more eloquent, spread renown, clarify doubts in ancient texts, and sometimes uncover new ideas. This happens when a secret idea imparted to a disciple by a teacher may be advanced by the disciple enthusiastically to win a debate! Discussion is therefore useful and necessary for the physicians and the disciples. The discussions which appear often in Caraka Saṃhitā (CS) are excellent examples of how the disciples were benefitted by the central theme identified by Ātreya, the diverse points of view expressed by disciples freely during the discussions and summing up by Ātreya, which reconciled different points of view at the conclusion of the discussion.

Practical training: Ayurvedic teachers were deeply conscious of the crucial role of practical experience in a physician's training. Suśruta likened a physician without practical training and experience to a one-winged bird, helpless, and an object of pity (Figure 3). In saluting an ideal physician, Vāgbhaṭa highlighted "mastery in practical arts" as one of the essential qualities. Caraka also mentions in several places "skill in the use of hand" (kṛtahastatā) as an important and essential part of a physician's armamentarium. The disciple therefore had plenty of opportunities for practical training during his life in the āśrama. In the collection and identification of herbs, preparation and storage of formulations, assisting the teacher-physician during domiciliary visits, performance of procedures and serving as a virtual apprentice during his years as a disciple, the Āśrama period was notable for the stress on acquisition of practical skills and experience.

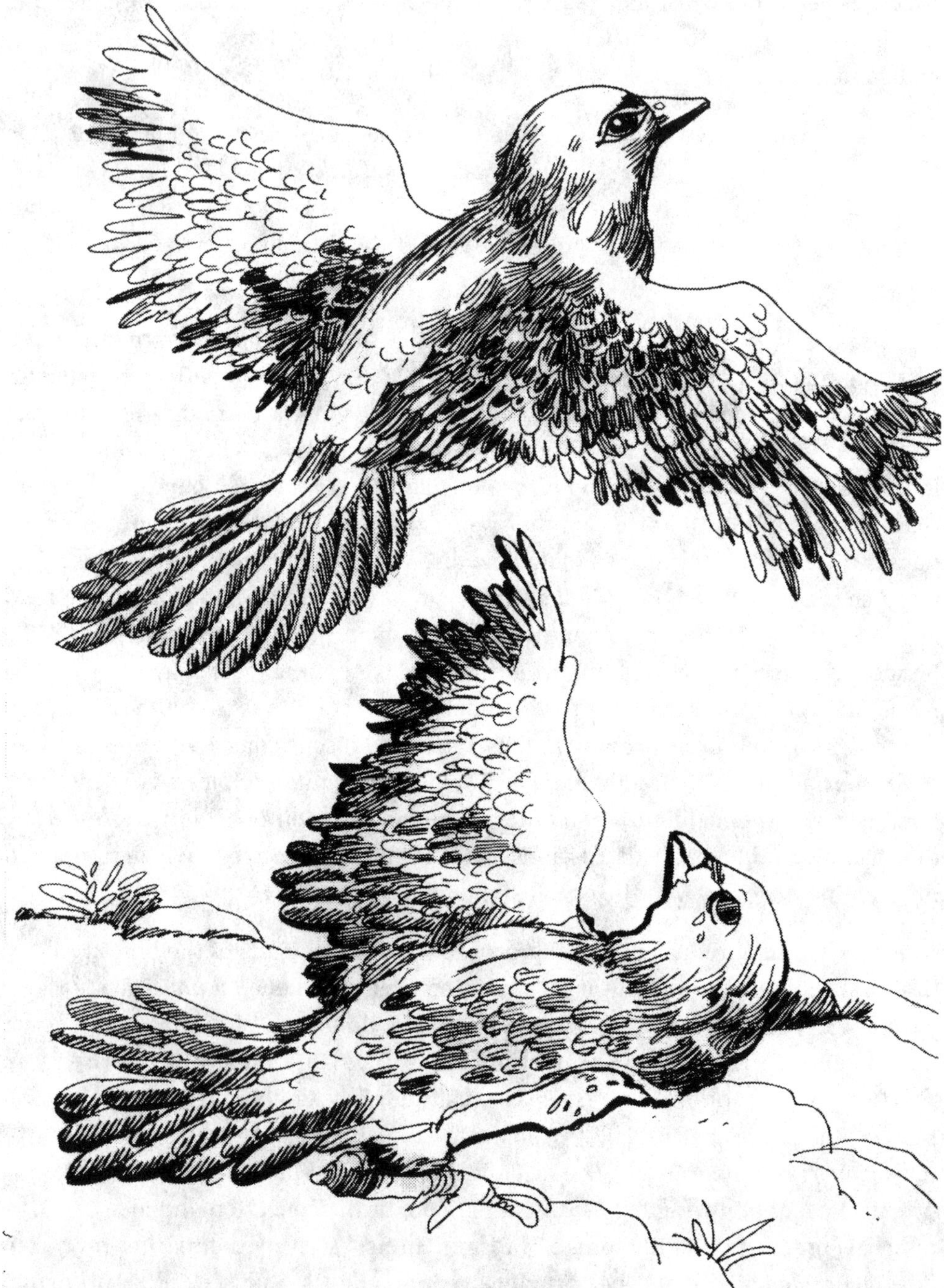

Figure 3*: *One winged bird

Note: Training in theory and practice are equally indispensable for a physician; training limited to one would cripple him like a one-winged bird.

Conclusion of training: The conclusion of training was not fixed based on a predetermined number of years in the Āśrama. The decision to conclude the training of a physician when he would be safe to practice medicine on his own on the public, was made by the teacher, who had personally supervised the training, known his professional knowledge, skill and character first hand. On the basis of the teacher's assessment, a physician had to get the permission from the King's officer before he could start practice on his own.

Special training in surgery: Suśruta Saṃhitā (SS) bears testimony to the principle that a surgeon should be a physician with the added skill to do surgical intervention. This would explain the authority of SS for the physician and surgeon even 17 centuries after its redaction by Nāgārjuna. Though no clear descriptions are available on the combined or sequential training in medicine and surgery in Āśrama, it would be reasonable to suppose that at some point, when a disciple had gained above average knowledge and skill in medicine and had shown aptitude for a surgical career, the preceptor would send him to a "Dhanvantari school" for specialized training in surgery.

Saṃhitā (SS) opens with a scene, where Kāśirāja Divodāsa revered as an incarnation of Lord Dhanvantari receives a group of students including Suśruta, who had approached him to learn surgery. It is tempting to speculate whether this was typical of what happened elsewhere in India too in the training of surgeons. The students headed by Suśruta, who appeared before Kāśirāja Divodāsa were already physicians because, on learning from them that their intent was the study of Āyurveda, Divodāsa asked them, "Which branch of Āyurveda do you wish to learn?" This question implied specialization in one of the branches of Āyurveda as anyone Āyurveda–illiterate could not specialize in one branch of Āyurveda. Similarly, physicians with basic training in Āyurveda and special interests would have gone to other great preceptors to receive specialized training in the treatment of poisoning (agada), children's diseases (kaumārabhṛtya), and so on. This was an ancient anticipation of what happens in the present-day graduation and postgraduate specialization in medicine.

Training of physicians in a University

When Suśruta and Caraka were at the zenith of their professional achievement, Takṣaśilā (Taxila in Pakistan) was renowned all over India and Asia as a great center of learning. It was reputed to be the oldest international university as it dated back to 8th century BCE and drew students numbering 10,000 from all over India and Asia and prided in having 2,000 teachers. It had outstanding faculty in many subjects, which included vedic studies, linguistics, medicine, military science, law, and skills such as archery and hunting. Its faculty is believed to have included Kauṭilya or Cānakya, Caraka, and Pāṇini; Jīvaka, an alumnus of Takṣaśilā, became the personal physician of the Buddha and Emperor Bimbisāra – son of Chandragupta Maurya. Takṣaśilā shone brightly as a beacon in higher learning until the fifth century CE, when it was destroyed by the nomadic Huns.

While we do not have a detailed account of the educational programs and practices in Takṣaśilā, we are fortunate to have vivid information about Jīvaka's training as a physician in Takṣaśilā and subsequent career. As Jīvaka and Takṣaśilā shared mutual immortality, his career as a physician could be considered to reflect, although indirectly, the quality of training for physicians in the great University.

Jīvaka was born as an orphan in Pāṭalīputra, but was found and reared as a prince in the palace by Abhaya, son of Emperor Bimbisāra. A precocious boy, he decided to make himself a top physician and, as a teenager, travelled all the way to Takṣaśilā for getting training. Ācārya Ātreya accepted him as a disciple because Jīvaka impressed him instantly by his sharp intelligence, candour, and enthusiasm. As he had no money to pay the fees, he took part time service in lieu, as this was an accepted practice in Takṣaśilā. He excelled in studies and outdid all his fellow disciples. After seven years of hard training, the teacher gave him a test, which involved going around Takṣaśilā campus for 16 miles in four days and coming up with a plant, which was useless for medical treatment. Jīvaka did the circumambulation as commanded and returned empty handed. On telling the teacher, "Sir, I could find no plant in my search, which had no medical application," he was pleased and declared him passed. As Jīvaka was poor, the teacher even gave him money to go back to Rajagir.

On his way back, Jīvaka treated a rich merchant's wife, who had suffered from headache for several years, which did not respond to treatment by senior physicians. Jīvaka treated her by a self-made naśya and gave her instant relief. Back in Rajagir, he did a trephining of the skull of a rich patient, who had been given a week to live by the doctors. Jīvaka removed two worms through the trephined hole from the brain and cured the patient. He successfully operated an Emperor Bimbisāra for anal fistula. He was accepted by Buddha as his personal physician, which, as an ardent devotee of the Blessed One, Jīvaka accepted with alacrity. A busy doctor, he used to charge high fees from rich patients and gift all that he received to the Buddhist Sangha. In his personal, professional, and spiritual life, Jīvaka shone brilliantly and brought credit to his University and everlasting inspiration to his successors in India. Though the Jātaka literature contains a great deal about him and he is well known in Buddhist countries, he is hardly remembered in India, where his life and work were cast.

Training of Ayurvedic physicians; advances in the 20th century

Few would disagree that the stagnation and decline in Āyurveda had been relentless for a 1000 years, when the British established their colonial rule in India in the 18th century. The British rulers shared Macaulay's contempt for India's cultural heritage of which Āyurveda was an important part. Deprived of State support for centuries during Islamic rule which preferred Unani, British authorities refused to accept Āyurveda as anything but herbal therapy. Takṣaśilā and Naḷanda long vanished, Gurukula system in total disarray, professional organizations non-existent, support from the Government lacking, Āyurveda faced a crisis of existence in the 19th century. A few pioneers here and there such as Gananath Sen in Kolkata, P S Varier in Kottakkal and Lakṣmīpati in Chennai kept the flame alive by their prodigious effort. A brief look at the experience in training physicians in Kottakkal is instructive as a case study.

Trained in the Gurukula system, Sanskrit scholar, connoisseur of performing arts and a brilliant physician, P S Varier was also open to modernity. He apprenticed himself to Dr Varghese – a physician trained in modern medicine - for three years and, without compromising his immense pride in Āyurveda, took note of many areas in the practice and teaching of medicine, where Āyurveda could benefit from adopting western methods. The manufacture of Ayurvedic drugs of high quality in full compliance with ancient formulae was a daring example of this East-West encounter in Kottakkal, though it had been preceded by one or two enterprises in Bengal such as N N Sen and Company of Kolkata in 1884. What is important for us is the initiative of P S Varier for the training of Ayurvedic physicians. As early as 1910, he wanted to establish a "Pāṭhaśāla" (school) to teach an "Aryavaidyan." The proposed rules for the institution published in "Dhanvantari" dated 10 December 1910 included a four-year course; anatomy, physiology, surgery, and drug manufacturing, besides Aṣṭāṅgahṛdaya, Sanskrit, and attending on patients in the hospital. But, support for the proposal was weak from the "affluent society" of Kerala and nil from the government in spite of the promotive effort of Varier's Arya Vaidya Samajam. He wrote movingly about the delay in Dhanvantari in January 1914.

> Knowledgeable vaidyans are growing fewer in number. And even those who are considered knowledgeable now, compared to the old-time vaidyans, we will have to accept that the present day vaidyans do not deserve to be called vaidyans at all. If we make a close search, one or two might be seen to have learnt something from the worthwhile physicians of old. With the next generation, we cannot even hope

> to make any effort in this direction. So, there is no doubt at all that the first thing we should do is to establish a vaidyapāṭhaśāla. If the objective of this pāṭhaśāla is to be fulfilled, it is an indisputable fact that there must also be a hospital and a centre to process medicines attached to it. English medicine had taken us over completely. It had every imaginable kind of tool as well as assistance from the King. Not only do we not have any of these, we have to confess now that we do not even have basic knowledge. There is no need then to say what the future will be.[7]

The pāṭhaśāla was finally inaugurated on 14 January 1917 and never looked back. Today's illustrious cluster of institutions in Kottakkal including the Hospital, Industry, and Educational institutions grew out of the prolonged struggles against many odds in the early years of the 20th century. After independence, education in Āyurveda has expanded dramatically with government support at the under graduate and postgraduate level with a Central Council, which sets up and maintains the academic standards. The present curriculum for the BAMS degree consists of Āyurveda and a considerable amount of modern science and medicine, a trend which was foreseen 100 years ago.

References:

1. *CS Sūtra* 1: 32–40
2. *CS Vimāna* 8: 3–5
3. *CS Vimāna* 8: 7–9
4. *CS Vimāna* 8: 11–12
5. *CS Vimāna* 8: 13–14
6. *CS Vimāna* 8: 15
7. *A Life of Healing–A Biography of Vaidyaratnam P S Varier*. Gita Krishnankutty. Pages 111-112: 2001.

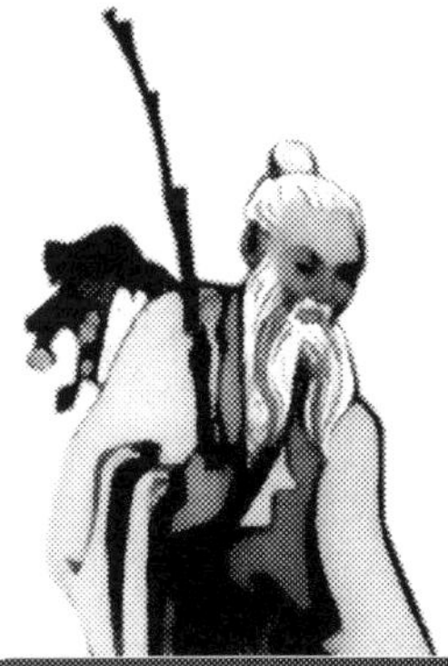

CHAPTER 16

A Science Initiative in Āyurveda (ASIIA)

Modern Science

The title may appear redundant to those who look upon Āyurveda as a science, which has been known, taught, and applied in therapeutics for many hundreds of years. The explanation is that the "Science" in the title refers to modern science, which appeared in Europe during renaissance, when a whirlwind gripped the human mind with unprecedented consequences in art, sculpture, and science. All these existed earlier, but the liberation of human spirit which renaissance witnessed brought about profound changes in the way they were practiced. Two specific examples would illustrate the changes which were transformational in medicine.

Anatomy was known and taught in Europe from the time of Hippocrates and a great deal of the structure of the human body was described by authorities including Aristotle and Galen. However, the anatomical descriptions, in common with the ancient descriptions of Suśruta, were not accurate. The wind of change in the 16th century produced a remarkable physician and anatomist – Andreas Vesalius – who studied human anatomy over several years by meticulous dissection and authored a masterly and authoritative book "De Humani Corporis Fabrica." Its attention to detail and accuracy of description had no precedent, which became the guiding principles of scientific endeavour ever since. The second example relates to function or physiology in the human body. A major subject in physiology is the circulation of blood, which had interested physicians from ancient times including especially, Galen. It was believed that blood was pumped out by the heart – that much was known – but the puzzle was how did blood return to the heart to be pumped out again? This defied an explanation and various theories like "invisible pores" in the heart had been advanced to explain the puzzle. It was left to William Harvey, a British physician of the 17th century to describe the circulation of blood accurately; that arteries and veins form a complete circuit, which starts in the heart and leads back to the heart by the regular contractions of the heart which drive the flow the blood. By this historic contribution to knowledge, Harvey established that scientific hypothesis would remain an aborted discovery as long as it does not graduate through experiment. Accurate observation and experiment remain the twin pillars of research in biology and medicine.

Heady with a spirit of new science in Europe, a Portuguese physician Garcia da Orta, came to Goa in the 16th century (Figure 1). He stayed on for 36 years and practiced medicine in Goa, where the Portuguese population was devastated by tropical diseases like cholera which even claimed Governors. Portuguese physicians were few in number, which obliged the authorities to make use of the medical resources of the "natives." Garcia took great interest in India's medicinal plants and their use in the treatment of various diseases. He wrote a famous book "Colloquies on the Simples and Drugs of India," which became a bestseller in Europe as Europeans had eyed India for long. They were drawn to its fabulous wealth and opportunity for plunder, but had been put off by the fear of tropical diseases. Garcia's book was the first and authentic introduction of the traditional medicine of India to the Europeans. The trail was picked up on a grander scale by the Dutch Governor of Kochi, Van Rheede, who was fascinated by the medicinal properties of plants on the Malabar Coast in the 17th century (Figure 2). Over a 30-year Odyssey, his team of over a hundred including field workers, herbalists, professors of botany, clergymen, artists, engravers, and an Ayurvedic physician – Itty Achuthan – laboured and produced a masterpiece – Hortus Malabaricus, which was published in 12 volumes in Latin from Amsterdam. It featured over 700 plants in four languages, exquisite illustrations and indications on their medicinal use (Figure 3). Garcia and Van Rheede started off a scientific revolution in taxonomy in India, which caught on rapidly as it involved many institutions and gave a strong impetus to research in medicinal plants. In the 20th century, medicinal plants attracted the attention of pharmacologists pioneered by Sir R N Chopra in Kolkata, who specifically sought to develop drugs from traditional sources for use in modern medicine (Figure 4). His effort inspired many scientists all over India and even institutes to develop drugs from medicinal plants. As a corollary, natural products chemistry flourished and continues to be pursued vigorously. Historically, it was inevitable that molecular biology would become the next biological science to lead studies in traditional medicine in India especially, Āyurveda.

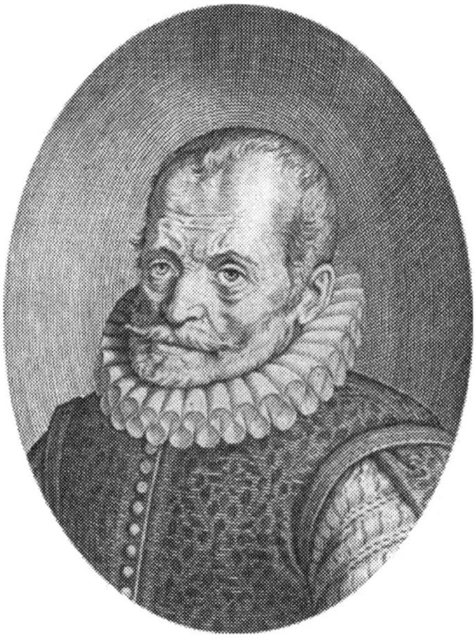

Figure 1: Garcia da Orta

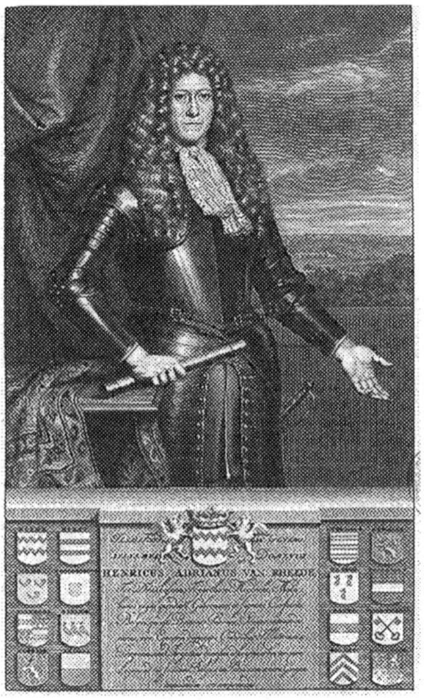

Figure 2: Van Rheede

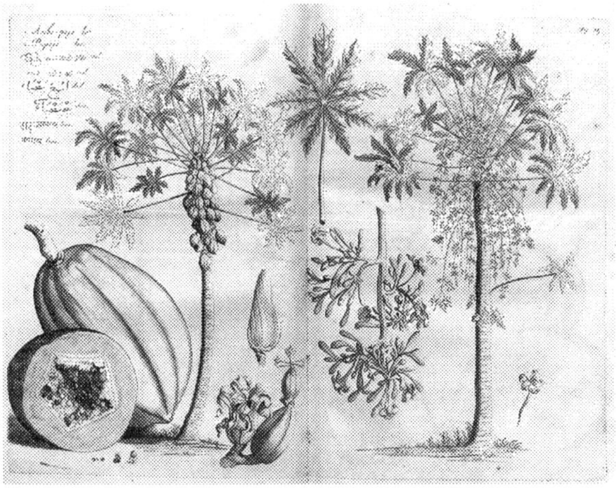

Figure 3: Plants from Hortus Malabaricus

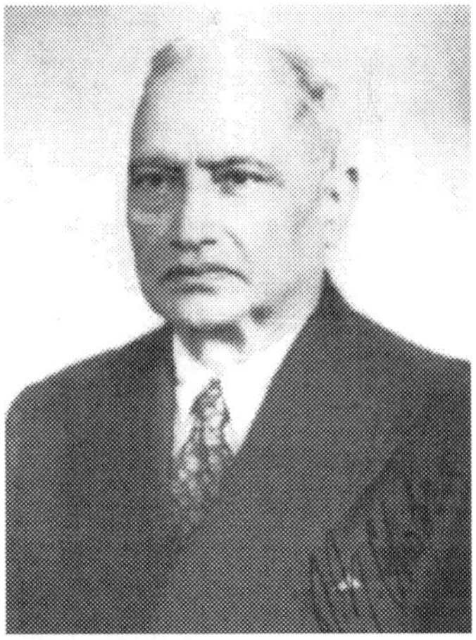

Figure 4: Sir R N Chopra

Status of research in Āyurveda

Though European science and Āyurveda began their encounter in the 16th century, scientific research in Āyurveda grew at a slow pace. Currently, Ayurvedic research falls under three broad categories:

- Medicinal plants: Herbal drugs;
- Clinical research; and
- Biomedical science.

The dominant category is without doubt herbal drugs and medicinal plants. As noted earlier, taxonomy and pharmacological studies based on medicinal plants have been pursued vigorously for over a century and India has a significant indigenous industry for herbal products, many departments in the universities working on medicinal plants, and government institutes devoted to medicinal plants and herbal drug development. The research output in terms of papers published from India in this segment is quite impressive. However, the fact remains that none of the plant derived drugs of the classical era - codeine, atropine, ephedrine, quinine, or emetine – emerged from India. Nor could Indian effort produce a "block buster" drug with global reach in the treatment of infectious or non-communicable diseases. This is admittedly an unsatisfactory situation which calls out for a diagnosis to be made, treatment prescribed, and worked for urgently.

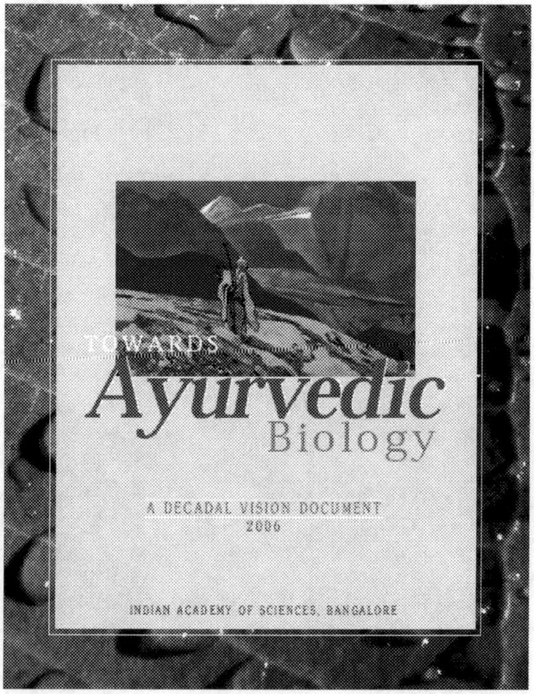

Figure 5: Towards Ayurvedic Biology; Decadal Vision Document of the Indian Academy of Sciences, 2006.

As far as the clinical research goes, the situation is complex. Most of what goes on in clinical research is, in fact, clinical trials including randomized, double-blind, controlled trials. However, Āyurveda does not subscribe to the concept of "controlled" trials, because it postulates the uniqueness of the doṣa-prakṛti of individuals, who cannot be grouped homogenously as "study" and control groups. Thanks to this difficulty which is shared by some other systems of traditional medicine, WHO suggested in 2000 CE a new set of guidelines for the clinical trial of drugs in traditional systems. These guidelines were liberal in so far as "randomized, double-blind, controlled trials" were no longer mandatory even though their supremacy as evidence remained undiminished. The liberalized guidelines included the patient being accepted as his/her own control and treatment as a "black box" consisting of poly herbal formulations, dietary regimen, and medical procedures being accepted without dissecting the box. Despite these liberalized guidelines, no clinical trials have been conducted, as far as known, in compliance with them in India.

In the third segment of research, applying basic sciences – mainly modern biology, immunology, biological chemistry – to research in Āyurveda, a beginning has been made through a science initiative only in recent years. This was anticipated by the Decadal Vision Document "Towards Ayurvedic Biology" published by the Indian Academy of Sciences in 2006 (Figure 5). The document drew the attention of Dr R Chidambaram, Principal Scientific Advisor (PSA) to the Government of India as it fitted well in the "Directed Basic Research" scheme launched by his office. Thanks to the support extended by his office and the Department of Science and Technology (DST), several research projects were carried out in the first decade of the "Science Initiative in Āyurveda," which was reviewed recently.[1] The main difficulties in advancing research in the new field of Ayurvedic Biology are outlined below:

Identification of study questions: Ayurvedic biology is biology qualified by Āyurveda. The qualification consists of a cue derived from Ayurvedic concepts, procedures, or putative effects of products or procedures. Identification of the cues requires clinical experience or deep understanding of Āyurveda; the biological research based on the cues would require knowledge and experience in designing experiments, use of sophisticated instrumentation and the skill and experience to interpret the findings correctly. To illustrate, consider doṣa-prakṛti in Āyurveda which indicates the constitutional type of an individual. This is highly important because it is fixed at the moment of conception in utero and is unalterable; it determines one's predisposition to diseases and an individual's response to treatment.

Traditionally, a physician would look at the physical, mental, and behavioural traits of a given patient and identify his prakṛti based on the traits - prakṛti connection listed in classical texts such as CS and AH. While this practice seems to have worked well for the physicians, it would not be accepted currently as "evidence" for the classification of individuals. As a matter of fact, 30 years ago, science did not have the tools or methods to do genotyping to classify individuals and populations. However, advances in the techniques of molecular biology have placed in the hands of investigators reliable methods and tools to study a variety of markers such as SNPs and determine whether doṣa specific markers exist in individuals. This is merely an example of how modern biology has been successfully employed to study the question of doṣa-prakriti.[2] There are many more questions, which would greet an eager scientist on the trail of Ayurvedic cues for biological research.

Designing experimental protocols on the basis of information in ancient texts: Even when the choice of formulations or procedures for research is confined to those figuring in the ancient texts recognized by the Ministry of AYUSH, the methods prescribed in them for the same formulation may not be identical. The synonyms used for plants, interpreting weights and measures, absence of elaborate details in the methods – required in today's protocol – pose many difficulties in writing an experimental protocol. An example is a study of the micro structure of Rasasindūra. The collaboration of a thoroughly professional Ayurvedic center is indispensable in undertaking this kind of research as they must make the rasasindūra samples with batch-to-batch consistency.[3] Projects in Ayurvedic Biology cannot succeed or give further cues for new lines of investigation unless a high level scientific institute and a research–friendly Ayurvedic center collaborate closely in the work. This study illustrates how rasasindūra made by Arya Vaidya Śala of Kottakkal according to ancient protocol was characterized by the state-of-the-art technique of XAFS in the Bhaba Atomic Research Centre, Mumbai.

Creating science - Āyurveda partnerships: Since the entry of European science in India in the 19th century, there has been virtually no interaction between scientists and Ayurvedic physicians. Even in the study of medicinal plants, the medicinal botanists and chemists work on their own with little role for the Ayurvedic physicians in their study. This "Do it alone" approach is self-defeating, as the research in numerous medicinal plants since independence has not produced any major drug in India, which had significant impact on therapeutics or commerce. Scientists deprive themselves of valuable, if not indispensable, inputs from the clinical experience with the use of drugs when they exclude Ayurvedic physicians from a project; conversely, Ayurvedic physicians impoverish themselves by not seeking active collaboration with scientists in investigating traditional procedures and drugs. An example of successful partnership was a study on the treatment of obesity by Basti (part of pañcakarma), which is traditionally done in Āyurveda. The procedure was planned and done in the Podar Hospital, Mumbai while the immunological and metabolic changes in the subjects during and after the procedure were done in The Advanced Centre for Treatment, Research and Education in Cancer (ACTREC) and Nair Hospital, Mumbai. The study showed that the subjects not merely lost weight significantly, but also their level of insulin–resistance causing pro-inflammatory cytokines, immunoglobulins and functional properties of T cells were significantly reduced as a result of Basti. Obesity is inflammatory in origin and basti obviously counters it.[4]

It seems apparent that in the absence of discovery-oriented or product-oriented research done jointly by scientific and Ayurvedic groups, India may not succeed in discovering a drug to prevent or treat major diseases such as, for example, a drug from medhyarasāyanas for dementias.

Overcoming skepticism among scientists and Ayurvedic physicians: The British rulers in India took the initiative in setting up hospitals, medical colleges, and over a dozen research institutions in medical science in India in the second half of the 19th and early 20th century, but they never gave encouragement to Āyurveda because it was regarded as herbal therapy. Unfortunately, Indians trained in the British-designed institutions followed suit and acquired the same prejudices regarding traditional knowledge and practices. On the other hand, Ayurvedic physicians – over 22,000 graduates being produced every year – are largely averse to science-based protocols being applied to Ayurvedic research on the ground that Āyurveda is "epistemologically" different; it has been practiced successfully for 5, 000 years; and it requires no "validation" by science. Unless, these harmful and ignorant views are eschewed by both sides, projects in Ayurvedic biology cannot succeed.

Lack of financial support: Announcements of liberal support for scientific research in Āyurveda are regularly made by politicians and senior administrators, but the reality is very different. Funds for research in Āyurveda are miniscule and there are also doubts whether what little is available is spent optimally. The relative success of the ASIIA scheme is entirely due to the far-righted support extended to it by the office of the Principal Scientific Advisor (PSA), Government of India, when no agency or organization was willing to even consider it. Until the scheme was taken over by DST as a Task Force in Ayurvedic Biology, even the future of ASIIA was uncertain!

Task Force in Ayurvedic Biology

ASIIA supported by the PSA's office was a novel experiment in the field of Ayurvedic research. Unlike earlier efforts, which focused on herbal drugs almost exclusively, here was an attempt to use the state-of-the-art tools of biology, immunology, and physical sciences to understand the basic concepts, procedures, and mechanistic basis of the action of procedures and products by partnering institutions of science and Āyurveda. In the first three years, the Science initiative supported five research projects, which drew reputed scientists and Ayurvedic physicians as Principal

Investigators from institutions across India. The progress of the new scheme caught the eye of the DST, who set up a "Task Force in Ayurvedic Biology" as a regular mechanism for promoting research in this nascent field of inter-disciplinary search. The Task Force has a sharply focused agenda because it excludes research in herbal drugs and clinical trials for safety and efficacy and confines itself to the support of research which employs basic sciences to investigate study questions in Āyurveda. It has received the growing attention of the scientific and Ayurvedic fraternities and yielded substantial publications in genomics, immunology, and materials science in so far as they impinge on Āyurveda. Metaphorically, the published results of these studies resemble new sprouts here and there in an age-old tree, which will before long be covered with fresh sprouts all over!

References:

1. *Ayurvedic Biology: The First Decade*. Proceedings of Indian National Science Academy. Vol. 82, No. 1, March 2016.
2. Determinants of Prakṛti, the Human Constitution Types of Indian Traditional Medicine and its Correlation with Contemporary Science. Harish Rotti, Ritu Raval, Suchitra Anchan, Ravishankara Bellampalli, Sameer Bhale, Ramachandra Bharadwaj, Balakrishna K Bhat, Amrish P Dedge, Vikram Ram Dhumal, G G Gangadharan, T K Girijakumari, Puthiya M Gopinath, Periyasamy Govindaraj, Swagata Halder, Kalpana S Joshi, Shama Prasada Kabekkodu, Archana Kamath, Paturu Kondaiah, Harpreet Kukreja, K L Rajath Kumar, Sreekumaran Nair, S N Venugopalan Nair, Jayakrishna Nayak, B V Prasanna, M Rashmishree, K Sharanprasad, Kumarasamy Thangaraj, Bhushan Patwardhan, Kapaettu Satyamoorthy, and Marthanda Varma Sankaran Valiathan. *Journal of* Āyurveda *and Integrative Medicine*, 5(3):167 - 75, (2014).
3. Investigating structural aspects to understand the putative/claimed non-toxicity of the Hg-based Ayurvedic drug Rasasindhūra using XAFS. Nitya Ramanan, Debdutta Lahiri, Parasmani Rajput Ramesh Chandra Varma, A Arun, T S Muraleedharan, K K Pandey, Nandita Maiti, S N Jha, and Surinder M Sharma. *Journal of Synchrotron Radiation*, 22, 1233 – 1241, (2015).
4. Immunological and metabolic responses to a therapeutic course of *Basti* in obesity. Urmila Thatte, Shubhada Chiplunkar, Supriya Bhalerao, Aditi Kulkarni, Raman Ghungralkar, Falguni Panchal, Shamal Vetale, Pradeep Teli, Dipti Kumbhar, and Renuka Munshi, *Indian Journal of Medical Research*, 142(1), 53 – 62, (2015).

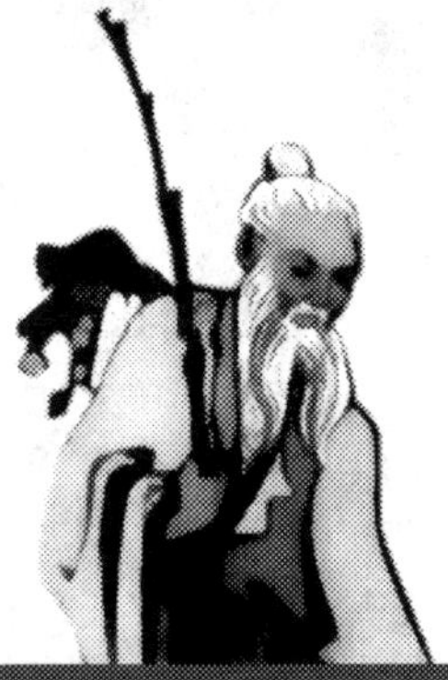

CHAPTER 17

Musings on Āyurveda

I. Philosophical

1. Nature

What is nature? When Kālidāsa wrote "maranam prakṛtiḥ śarīriṇām" (death is the nature of embodied beings) he implied nature as the primal condition from which life evolves and to which it returns. Sāṅkhya philosophy viewed prakṛti as the original, undifferentiated source of the physical universe with three latent guṇas – sattva, rajas, and tamas. Poet and artists had their own definitions. Against these variegated ideas, Āyurveda took an overarching view, which identified prakṛti as a product of svabhāva (Inmate disposition), Īśvara (Providence), kāla (Time), yadṛcchā (Chance), niyati (Fate), and pariṇāma (Evolution). Each is unique and integral to the making of nature.[1]

Svabhāva (Innate disposition): Is the natural state or constitution termed prakṛti specific to individuals? There are three main types of designated doṣa prakṛtis in Āyurveda – vāta, pitta, and kapha, which determine the events taking place in the body and its responses to external stimuli. Doṣa prakṛti is determined in Ayurvedic practice according to body and mental traits, which are listed in ancient texts. Prakṛti in relation to the body is a living concept.

Īśvara (Providence): In the present context, Īśvara is not the deity we worship but providence which is synonymous with the beneficence of nature. It is not limited to mountains, rivers, fauna, and flora, which are marked by powers of healing; it has provided an inherent tendency to heal from the life molecule DNA to organs, and instilled love and affection in parents to nurture their offspring. In the absence of this beneficence, survival of species, leave aside evolution, would come to a stop.

Kāla (Time): Is the constant background and determinant of a physician's endeavour. Diseases affecting children and elderly, inflammation progressing to suppuration, healing of fractures and wounds, growth of foetus in utero and countless other events in life are united by the thread of time. Ayurvedic classics are full of references to cycles day and night, procession of seasons in a year, fluctuations in rasas of vegetables with stages of ripening, and adverse effect of seasons on herbs and their use in therapy. While, the pañcabhūta doctrine of Āyurveda sought to identify the elements of the body with the constituents of the universe, the theory of adjusting life style to the seasons (ṛtucarya) represented a parallel endeavor to seek harmony between the microcosm and macrocosm during cyclical changes of seasons.

Yadṛcchā (Chance): Chance is defined as something which happens without an obvious cause. The subject of cause and effect had been debated in India from ancient times, echoes of which can be heard in CS. Though, the final view seemed to favour causality, an acasual view continued to have adherents. This was because no cause would be found for many events, which occurred in nature as well as in the body. Unseasonal weather, foetal abnormalities, attacks by wild animals, and many other conditions, which confronted a physician, had no apparent cause and Āyurveda was obliged to give space to an acausal domain or chance side by side with the cause and effect domain.

Āyurveda attached importance to chance because the unexpected course of diseases, unexpected recoveries despite grave prognosis, unexpected deaths of patients despite excellent treatment, and other clinical events made a profound impression on physicians. While the debate on the causal vs acausal was not settled, a practical test evolved to define the nature of a clinical event. If a man slipped and fell and suffered bruises, that would be an accident, a chance event; however, if he sustained a head injury, became comatose and died, that would be the effect of past karma. This practical test assigned a due place for chance and karma in human life to satisfy the advocates of acausal and causal aspects of events.

Niyati (Fate): From yadṛcchā and acausal, we are now face to face with karma and destiny. The law of karma is deeply engraved on the Indian mind and the belief that past deeds must bear fruit for everyone is widely held. The adverse turn of a patient's illness and questions of his life span often haunt a physician. If his life span is predetermined, what would expert treatment or invocations avail? Could the vigorous and expert treatment by the physician nullify the effect of karma and save the patient? This is a dilemma, which defies a clear answer. Caraka took the middle ground. If, past deeds of the patient have accumulated a certain force, the present deeds of the patient and physician done jointly must generate a force too; if the negative force from the past is overwhelming, the treatment may fail; on the other hand, if the force generated by the cooperative effort of the patient and physician is superior to the effect of past deeds, the patient would recover. This is a doctrine, which encourages hope and inspires effort.

Pariṇāma (Evolution): Āyurveda is based on the basic doctrine of pañcabhūta, which postulates that the universe and all its parts including the human body are composed of the same five elements – ether, air, fire, water, and earth. It raises the question, where did the elements originate? How did they become the countless parts of the universe of stupendous diversity? What would happen to them? Would they die like the human body? How did consciousness (cetana) arise in non-living elements? These topics were of great interest in the Āśramas and we hear echoes of discussions on these subjects in CS. The discussions led to a scheme, which posited that in the beginning, when the universe did not exist there was nothing but an undifferentiated, indefinite, primordial existence within which were three latent forces of sattva, rajas, and tamas (avyakta). Then, a sudden disturbance or imbalance in the state of the three forces took place, a chance event which is neither predictable, nor controllable. This was followed by a cascade of events – Avyakta, buddhi; ahaṅkāra and so on until the cascade ended in the immense diversity of the universe, all this accounting for 24 stages or "tatvas." In good time, the universe would dissolve into the original Avyakta and start the cosmic cycle again. This theory advanced by Caraka is hailed as the original Sāṅkhya doctrine – preceding the classical version of Īśvarakṛṣṇa, confirming Caraka's claim to immortality as a philosopher–physician. The doctrine claimed that the world in some undifferentiated or differentiated form was always there and would always be there.

In the Ayurvedic vision, man is part of the nature. Nowhere did Āyurveda draw evidence from nature of a sovereign power, which was identified with God. The fundamental stuff of man and the universe is one composed by five bhūtas. As a part of nature, man owes his existence to a continuous interchange between himself and the natural environment. The interchange involves eating food and breathing air, which are lifeless things. But, the lifeless becomes alive in the body and this bio-transition occurs due to the incorporation of consciousness (cetana), which is synonymous with self. The Ayurvedic view of the human body is a far cry from the Cartesian view that a particular collection of bones, muscles, veins, and other structures put together would move by the arrangement of organs like a machine in the absence of self. (Caraka)

2. Eternal Āyurveda

Āyurveda is without beginning (anāḍi) and is perennial, says Caraka. It is eternal because the tradition (śaśvata) of healing in Āyurveda has neither a beginning nor an end. Beasts, when they are ill, seek out plants in their neighbourhood and chew on them, which they never do otherwise. This was recorded in a famous hymn of the Atharvaveda.

Varaho veda vīrudham nakulo veda bheṣajīm
Sarpā gandharva yā vidustha asma avase huve
Yāh suparṇa āngirasordivyā yā rakhaṭo viduḥ
Vayorsi hamsā yā viduryāśca sarve pathaṭrnah.[2]

I call upon the healing herbs of the Angirasas known by kites, the divine herbs known by raghats (probably bees) and the plants known by swans to protect us.

Healing practices are therefore as old as life. Āyurveda, whose core consists of healing, had neither a founder nor a date of birth, but it saved from diseases and suffering, living beings whose elemental composition of five bhūtas is permanent. Moreover, Āyurveda dealt with substances – animate and inanimate – whose qualities were inherent in them according to the law of inherence (samavāya) which is again eternal. As one probes deeper, it soon becomes apparent that there was never a time, when life and intellect did not exist as they are latent in the original state of avyakta in the cycle of evolution (pariṇāma). Health and disease, happiness and misery, substances and their properties are no more than products of the evolutionary cycle, which is also eternal. Āyurveda did not arise out of nothing, but represented a channel in the eternal flow of nature.[3] It is in this sense that Āyurveda is eternal.

II. Ethical

1. Four pursuits

Human life has four objects which are dharma, artha, kāma, and mokṣa. Dharma is often identified with righteousness, but there is no absolute good or evil for all human beings at all times. In discussing the relative nature of dharma, Mahabharata famously declared that the "Essence of dharma is hidden in a dark cave" (dharmasya tatvam nihitam guhāyām). Dharma is what determines one's proper attitude to all living beings and proper mental and physical response to events and situations. This would involve truthfulness, offering hospitality to guests, a soldier dying for his country while killing enemies or a saint laying down his life to save a life.

The second pursuit, wealth, is indispensable to keep the body and soul together. It is equally necessary for the society to survive as it needs wealth to build hospitals, schools, organize farming and many other constructive activities. Money is also necessary for humanity to find leisure for cultural activities and save itself from back breaking drudgery. But, the acquisition of wealth must be governed by dharma.

The third object, kāma, is the enjoyment of sense pleasures, which covers a vast range. Here again, the pursuit should be controlled by dharma lest it should end up in out and out hedonism.

The fourth object mokṣa, is the final emancipation of man who, in essence, is spirit and cannot be content or at peace permanently with worldly experiences alone.

However, no matter how varied or difficult the pursuit of the four objects may be, good health is indispensable for its success. The four objectives – puruṣārthas – rest on a healthy mind in a healthy body. Moreover, diseases could rob the individual of well-being or even destroy his life. Āyurveda which protects the health of the healthy and counters the diseases of the sick is the gift of gods for suffering humanity.[4] (Caraka)

2. A measure of life

Āyurveda is a measure of life, wholesome/unwholesome, happy and unhappy. Hailed by savants as the most meritorious among Vedas, because it bodes well for life here and hereafter, Āyurveda is concerned with life in its entirety involving body, sense organs, mind, and self. But, what do the terms wholesomeness (hita), happiness (sukha), and their opposites mean in defining Āyurveda?[5] What were the traits of wholesomeness and happiness, which lent themselves for measurement? According to Āyurveda, wholesomeness signifies good will for all living beings, absence of covetousness, truthfulness, tranquility, fore thought, constant vigilance, ability to combine virtue, wealth and enjoyment harmoniously, respect for the savants, devotion to knowledge, rejoicing in the company of the old, self-control, charity, fondness for knowledge and spirituality, attention to this world and the next, intelligence, memory of one's past, and true identity – which are the characteristics of wholesomeness; unwholesomeness consists of traits that are opposed to what are listed above. Notice that the traits in the list are largely moral traits and they are mentioned ahead of personal traits of happiness which follow.

Happiness includes the absence of physical and mental illness, youthful strength, energy and manliness, good reputation, knowledge, strong sense organs, affluence, many sided achievements, and freedom to move as he likes. In contrast to wholesomeness, the attributes under happiness are individual traits. Āyurveda seeks to measure life in both aspects – moral as well as individual – which make life whole. Excellence confined to one domain would make life unbalanced. Āyurveda also recognises that the ultimate measure of life is death known by many different and suggestive names such as svabhāva (returning to one's self) and nirodha (annihilation). (Caraka)

3. A look within

A melancholy fact of modern life is the number of young students, aspiring actors, and ambitious entrepreneurs take their lives out of frustration, depression, and a growing feeling of being "fed up." Most of them are intelligent, hardworking, and highly aspirational. They share big dreams and are driven by vaulting plans and frenetic activity from the moment they wake up in the morning. Some struggle relentlessly, brave the headwind, overcome every obstacle and proceed to the high table and attain glory. For every hero who succeeds, there would be hundreds who fall by the wayside and are condemned to a feeling of unease and emptiness, frustration and psychosomatic disorders. Is there a way to join aspiration and hard work with a healthy mind and body? Is there a way to do work that matters and make a lasting impact and, at the same time, remain master of oneself?

This is not easy, when we are constantly bombarded by messages on what we should eat, how we should look, what we should read, how we should make a fortune quickly, and how to get a doctorate painlessly. The messages have a numbing effect on the mind and, by and by, lead to a situation where our mind is mortgaged and is filled with a jumble of ideas, ambitions, and hopes of other people. We do not stop for a moment to ask whether these constant assaults on our mind are worth anything at all. This look within, a moment of introspection, is the first step in getting to know ourselves and retaking possession of our mind. This would also mark the start of gaining control over ourselves and being truly free.

Introspection is not an elaborate, esoteric, or risky procedure. It is better to keep it low profile and build it into the fabric of our daily life. Listen to Vāgbhaṭa;[6]

> He, who is always aware of how his days and nights are spent, will never know sorrow.

Significantly, in the previous verse, the sage had commended;

> Compassion to living beings, charity, self-restraint, and identifying others' adversity as ours; as the hallmark of good conduct.[7]

The habit of introspection holds the key to understanding ourselves and gaining freedom from societal conditioning.

4. Practice of Medicine: Prime motivation

Practice of medicine dates back to the mists of antiquity. Perhaps its earliest version is seen among tribal people, where a folk healer is the only source of medical assistance. Folk medicine is still in vogue in large parts of India and consists of rituals, chants, and the use of herbal remedies. The traditional healer was chosen as per tribal custom and the community took care of his needs. Tribal custom might also oblige the patient to offer a gift to the healer, but this was not compulsory. For the folk healer, his practice of medicine was a sacred duty to which he was called by the tribal community. There was no question of a choice by an individual.

In the time of Atharvaveda, we hear about "hundreds of physicians" (bhiṣaks) and roving communities of physicians. There were communities based on their occupation, where practice was transmitted from one generation to the next and the practitioners followed the same customs, beliefs, and procedures approved by the community. Motivation and individual choice of a medical career played little role in the training of physicians.

By the time of the Buddha, there is plenty of evidence that individual choice of a physician's career existed in Takṣaśilā and physicians practiced medicine on their own and not as part of community service. Jīvaka - Buddha's legendary physician used to treat patients for a fee and donate the fees he received to the Saṃgha. Caraka denounced fraudulent physicians for false pretenses, malpractice, and chicanery.

In Jīvaka's seeking admission for a physician's training in Takṣaśilā under Ātreya, Caraka's description of students seeking admission under preceptors in Aśramas and the account of Suśruta and his fellow students approaching Kāśirāja Divodāsa for training in surgery, we have early records of individual choice by young students for a physician's career. What were their motivations for choosing the ancient profession? From Kāśirāja Divodāsa's exhortation to the young students, we get glimpses of what appealed to them. He stressed that Āyurveda was of divine origin as the original text of hundred thousand verses composed by Brāhma was subsequently shortened into eight sections; it offers options to study the science of life or science which promotes long life; or surgery which treats emergencies like severe injuries caused by wild animals and gives immediate results; and it offers high repute, generous income, and a place in heaven in after life.

The relative importance of the factors mentioned by Kāśirāja Divodāsa has evolved over many centuries since Suśruta's life time. Few would be motivated by divine origin, puranic stories of head transplantation or a place in heaven, but high repute and generous income continue to be powerful incentives for choosing a medical career even today. The incentives for choosing a physician's career have increased massively in the 20th century all over the world, thanks to the unprecedented expansion of medical and surgical services, heavy input of science and technology and the influence of health care industry. The challenge is how to keep the focus on the humanitarian aspect of medicine, while technology and industry tend to obscure it.

Caraka was conscious of the central role of the patient in Āyurveda and commented:

> A physician should consider all patients as his own sons and safeguard them from illness. Āyurveda was bequeathed by great sages for upholding righteous living and wellness, not for seeking wealth or enjoyment. The one, who practices medicine only for human welfare and not for earning money or enjoyment, ranks far above those who practice for money. The physician, who is moved by compassion as the supreme incentive for service to patients triumphs, accomplishes the four objectives of life and attains sublime happiness.[8]

III. Biomedical

1. Consciousness and the foetus

The paternal and maternal origins of the development of hard and soft tissues in the body are well known and recognized in Āyurveda. Hard and soft tissues are visible and their abnormalities are detectable by an observer. But, the developing foetus is more than hard and soft tissues, because it also comprises consciousness or soul, which is not visible to the naked eye. It is the entry of consciousness through the vehicle of the mind, into the foetus, which triggers the pulsations of the heart. As the heart of the foetus beats in synchrony with the mother's heart, the mother's body at this time has two hearts beating simultaneously within. This is the likely reason, why the mothers express special and unusual likes and dislikes for food, clothes, seeing certain animals, and so on. These are the desires of the foetus finding expression in the mother and hence the mandate to fulfill the desires, lest failure to do so should hurt the foetus.[9]

But, how does consciousness enter the foetus through the tissue barriers posed by the mother and the foetus? It is consciousness or soul (ātman) which activates the sensory and motor organs, breathing, blinking of eyes and presides over knowledge, intellect, life span, and sense of pleasure and pain. Souls transmigrate among humans, animals, and gods according to the law of Karma.[10] Though, soul is too subtle to be visible to the physical eyes, it is accessible to the eyes of higher knowledge and penance. Passing through a magnifying glass to burn fuel, the rays of the sun are not seen; similar is the unseen entry of the soul, into the foetus in the womb.[11]

2. Epidemics as an equaliser

Diseases are conditioned by doṣas, which influence the doṣa-specific predisposition to diseases, severity illness, and the individual's response to treatment. However, these doṣa-specific effects vanish, when an epidemic wipes out entire populations regardless of their constitutional types or doṣa prakṛiti, food habits, age, physical, and mental strength. How does one account for this phenomenon?

Though the victims may differ in many ways, the differences are subdued by serious derangements in their locale including its air, water, geography, and time. These could undergo major upheavals such as hot, chilly or dusty winds, pollution of water, flourishing of poisonous animals and mosquitoes, the flight of birds and people to other locations, and lastly, untimely and severe change of seasons.[12]

The root cause of these derangements in air, water, place, and time is unrighteousness (adharma), which could result from past or present actions of man. Unrighteousness of past and present actions is caused by imprudent conduct of persons resulting from erroneous judgment (prajñāparādha). This is marked by individuals resorting to particular actions in spite of the knowledge that the actions are harmful even to themselves. Kings and commoners are susceptible to this conduct with evil consequences to the entire kingdom or to smaller communities. It would seem that righteousness declines progressively age after age with corresponding decrease in the life span of human beings.[13]

To ward off epidemics and destruction of the habitat, rulers and the entire community are obliged to follow a code of righteous conduct.

3. Righteous conduct in preventive medicine

Everyone wishes to be happy with few exceptions. Academicians, physicians, politicians, policemen, students, and concert musicians focused on a career have the ultimate aim as happiness. They struggle, brave hardships, and endure insults to attain their much-sought aim of happiness. In the anxiety and impatience to move up quickly, they may be tempted time and again to take shortcuts or deviations, which may appear inconsequential. Therein, begins a slip down a greasy slope.

The academician lifts observations from the paper of a scientist only to be caught and charged with plagiarism; the physician tempted to do unlawful transplant operations to make a fortune ends up in jail; the politician finds himself behind the bars for bribery; policeman is dismissed for the death of an offender during custodial questioning; student debarred from taking examination for impersonation; and concert musician becomes an alcoholic, a shadow of his former self and an object of pity.

These are frequent events in contemporary India. Vāgbhaṭa would have seen the ancient prototypes of these misdemeanors and grieved over the frailty of human conduct and the burden of human bondage. In the above examples, the individuals driven by ambition were aware of their erroneous conduct, but could not exercise self-control. Imprudent or unethical conduct, even when a subject is aware of the error of impending action was well recognised in Āyurveda as prajñāparādha, which was believed to be a prominent cause of ailments. Many of these ailments would fall in the category of non-communicable or stress induced disorders in current phraseology. No medical therapy could be a substitute for righteous conduct.

4. Control of sense organs

The philosophical systems of India except lokāyata tend to agree that so long as mind follows the constant and endless chase of objects by our senses, tranquility would elude an individual. Bhagvadgīta refers to the powerful senses rocking the mind of even a spiritual seeker. Patañjali's yoga and many other yogic practices have practiced different methods to "suspend the operations of the mind" over many centuries and these methods were often accompanied by systematic efforts to control or suppress the sense organs. These efforts would take extreme forms such as prolonged fasting to chastise the taste organ, sticking thorns over the body to punish the touch organ, and so on. Everyone knows the experience of Gautama in Uruvela, where he joined five ascetics in a course of fasting and extreme penance and persisted so long that his body was reduced to skin and bones and he fell down unconscious. It was after a bitter struggle of six years that he realised the futility of extreme asceticism and torturing of senses for realising truth.

While insisting on a code of virtuous living, Āyurveda took the middle ground on the use of senses from the point of view of healthy living. In the first place, Vāgbhaṭa declared in no uncertain terms that "In the underuse, misuse, and overuse of time, sense objects and activity lie the roots of ill-health; appropriate use thereof safeguards good health."[14] He reiterated "Those who wish for happiness here and hereafter should keep their senses under control and rein in the mental urges of greed, jealousy, malice, rivalry, and passion."[15] The emphasis on restraint was loud and clear throughout the discussions on the use of senses in Āyurveda. It advocated a full life including the use of rejuvenant therapy and never favoured asceticism. The middle ground was expressed by Vāgbhaṭa in the dictum "Sense organs should neither be tormented nor pampered."[16]

5. Adverse drug reactions

Drugs are like nectar according to Āyurveda but, administered by the ignorant or negligent, they could become weapons of destruction.[17] A large part of the physician's training consists of learning how to determine the particular disequilibrium of doṣas in a patient and how to identify drugs for administration with properties exactly opposed to those of the deranged doṣas. Once identified, the dosage, frequency of administration, use of supplementary drugs, and medical procedures, such as pañcakarma too had to be decided by the physician keeping in mind the patient's strength and season. A lapse in any of these steps, especially in the choice of drugs, could give rise to complications, which may be serious and sometimes even fatal.

Āyurveda held that medical treatment which cures or palliates a disease but, at the same time, gives rise to another disease sooner or later is not genuine or authentic.[18] As the adverse drug reactions could be harmful or dangerous, it is incumbent on the physician to exercise extreme care in choosing appropriate drugs and planning the specific treatment for each patient so that adverse reactions to the drug may not turn into another disease.

6. A difficult surgical decision

A surgical procedure is mandatory in many situations such as serious wounds, fractures, intestinal obstruction, and stone in the bladder, cataract, and many others. These were dealt with in detail by Suśruta. However, he referred to another category of patients who posed a different and difficult question for the surgeon at a time, when there was no anesthesia and no means to carry out diagnostic and other investigations. These patients were seriously ill and carried a high risk of operative mortality. The surgeon was required to notify the royal officer of the procedure in advance and obtain permission for undertaking high risk operations. It was also known that death of a patient following or during operation could lead to a major punishment of the surgeon according to the Arthaśāstra. Under these circumstances, should the surgeon choose to intervene or opt for a safer course of inaction? Suśruta's advice was loud and clear. Said he "In the absence of surgery, death is certain, but surgery involves uncertainty. In that situation, a well-meaning physician should opt for surgery with the permission of authorities."[19] The current professional attitude toward high risk surgery is in line with Suśruta's advice.

IV. Pedagogical

1. Physicians in training lest they forget

Treating a sick individual, involves more than treating a disease with appropriate therapeutic measures. Successful practice of medicine would require a physician to have knowledge about the patient's locale, its fauna and flora, its residents and their food habits, life style and common diseases; about the basis of the choice of drugs as evident in the bhūta-based classification of drugs; acquisition of skill by constant practice; ability to instruct disciples and assistants and win their respect and cooperation; and above all, a noble personality, which instills confidence in the patient. This would make it imperative that his mental horizon is not limited to medicine, but also comprehends liberal arts and a feeling for the human condition.[20]

In the study of the scriptural texts of medicine, Āśrama traditions insist on learning by rote regardless of written texts being available. The practice of rote, strengthens memory, enhances the power of exposition and teaching but, in the absence of understanding the meaning of verses, learning by rote is futile. Study of texts without understanding the meaning is no better than an ass carrying a load of sandal wood without enjoying its fragrance.[21]

Mastering theory is not enough for a physician in training; practice is no less important. In the training of surgeons, a number of experimental models have been created for the trainee to practice all the basic surgical procedures and enhance skill in doing operations. If a physician is equally proficient in theory and practice, he would acquit himself well like a two-wheeled vehicle does on the battle field.

2. Echoes of a dialogue

Punarvasu, Ātreya propounded the view that the successful treatment of a sick patient calls for a quartet to be in place and each member of the quartet should fulfill four requirements. The quartet consisted of the physician, drug, attendant, and patient, who are fully capable of restoring the health of the patient. The requirements of the physician are profound knowledge of texts, mature experience in practice, practical skill, and cleanliness; the drug should be available in plenty, should be potent, amenable to preparation in many forms and stable; attendant should know bedside care, possess practical skill, loyalty and cleanliness; and the patient should have powers of recall, compliance with physician's instructions, courage and candor in recounting his illness to the physician. This aggregate of 16 requirements, if in place, bodes success in therapy, even though the physician's role is pre-eminent in view of his superior knowledge of medicine, authority, and role as a manager. His role is akin to that of a potter without whom clay, stick, wheel, and cord cannot make a pot. In the discussion on Punarvasu Ātreya's view on the medial quartet as the sheet anchor of therapeutics, Maitreya expressed his dissent as follows:

> It is well known to observers that some patients recover and some die, when the quartet is in charge of treatment and they fulfill the four requirements of each member. This would suggest that the therapeutic measures play little role in therapy; one could say that they are as useless as throwing a handful of water in a pond or scattering some dust on a heap of it. It is also observed that there are some patients who, in spite of the various deficiencies in the 16 requirements of the quartet, recover from illness, while others die. Treated or untreated, patients recover and die. Does this not suggest that therapy is no different from non-therapy?

Punarvasu Ātreya smiled and calmly responded, "Maitreya, you are mistaken! If, a patient dies in spite of treatment by a fully competent quartet, that does not mean treatment is ineffective in patients who are cured; conversely, if a patient recovers in spite of treatment by a quartet lacking in many requirements, that does not mean either that the therapy was useless and did not contribute to his recovery." Punarvasu Ātreya gave the illustration of a man who falls in a pit and tries to get out of it. While he may get out or get out with difficulty, a helping hand by someone would lighten his struggle. This helping hand is what medical therapy offers to a patient, who gets well quickly by the therapy administered by a complete quartet. Ātreya emphasized:

> It is true that patients may die, even when complete therapy is given by a fully competent quartet. This only confirms the fact that all diseases are not curable by therapeutic measures. It is equally true however, that curable diseases may not be cured in the absence of treatment. One should remember that therapeutics is ineffective in a moribund patient or in someone with an incurable disease. A good physician should examine all aspects of the patient and his disease with concentration like an archer ready to shoot a distant object and carry out his therapeutic measures in curable illnesses when success is sure to follow.[22]

The Ātreya–Maitreya dialogue gives us a glimpse into the way discussions (sambhāṣā) were held between a teacher and disciple in ancient Aśramas.

References

1. *SS Śārīra* 1: 11
2. *Atharva Veda* 8: 7: 23–24 [Text with Hindi translation by Pandit Sripad Damodar Satwalekar (1932) Paradi: Swadhyaya Mandal].
3. *CS Sūtra* 30: 27
4. *CS* 1:15
5. *CS Sūtra* 30: 24
6. *AH Sūtra* 2: 47
7. *AH Sūtra* 2: 46
8. *Cikitsā* 1.4: 55–62
9. *SS Śārīra* 3: 18
10. *SS Śārīra* 1: 16 – 17
11. *AH Śārīra* 1: 3
12. *CS Vimāna* 3: 6 – 7
13. *CS Vimāna* 3: 20 – 24
14. *AH Sūtra* 1: 19
15. *AH Sūtra* 4: 24
16. *AH Sūtra* 2: 29
17. *SS Sūtra* 3: 52
18. *AH Sūtra* 13: 16
19. *SS Cikitsā* 7: 28 – 29
20. *SS Sūtra* 4: 7
21. *SS Sūtra* 4: 4
22. *CS Sūtra* 10: 5

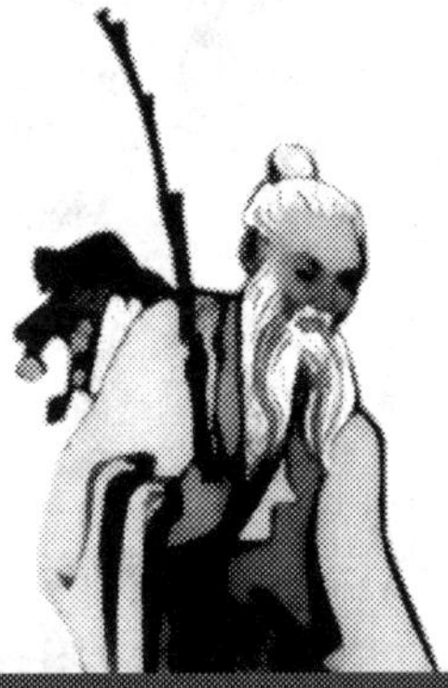

CHAPTER 18

Quotations

1. One who knows the text but is poor in practice gets confounded on seeing a patient; he is like a coward on the battle field.

2. One who is bold and dexterous but lacking in textual knowledge fails to win the approval of peers and risks capital punishment from the King. Having half knowledge, both are unequal to the job of a physician like a one-winged bird.

   यस्तु केवलशास्त्रज्ञः कर्मस्वपरिनिष्ठितः।
   स मुह्यत्यातुरं प्राप्य प्राप्य भीरुरिवाहवम्।।
   यस्तु कर्मसु निष्णातो धाष्ट्र्याच्छास्त्रबहिष्कृतः।
   स सत्सु पूजां नाप्नोति वधं चर्च्छति राजतः।।
   उभावेतावनिपुणावसमर्थौ स्वकर्मणि।
   अर्धवेदधरावेतावेकपक्षाविव द्विजौ।।
   Yastu kēvalaśāstrajña: karmasvaparinisṭhita:
   sa muhyatyāturaṃ prāpya prāpya bhīrurivāhavaṃ
   Yastu karmasu nisṇātō dhāṣṭyārcchāstrabahiṣkṛta:
   sa satsu pūjāṃ nāpnōti vadhaṃ carcchati rājata:
   Ubhāvētāvanipuṇāvasamarthau svakarmaṇi
   ardhavēdadharāvētāvēkapakṣāviva dvijau SS. Sū: 3. 48 - 50

3. He is healthy (svastha), whose doṣas, agnis, and the functions of dhātus and malas are in equilibrium; whose mind, intellect, and sense organs are bright and cheerful.

स्वस्थस्य रक्षणं कुर्यादस्वस्थस्य तु बुद्धिमान्।
क्षपयेद्बृंहयेच्चापि दोषधातुमलान् भिषक्।
तावद्यावदरोगः स्यादेतत्साम्यस्य लक्षणम्।।
Svasthasya rakṣaṇaṃ kuryādasvasthasya tu buddhimān
kṣapayēd bṛmhayēccāpi dōṣadhātumalān bhiṣak
tāvadyāvadarōga: syādētatsāmyasya lakṣaṇaṃ SS. Sū: 15 – 40

4. In a house that is architecturally perfect, clean, free from wind and sun, externally caused diseases and mental disorders would not occur.

प्रशस्तवास्तुनि गृहे शुचावातपवर्जिते।
निवाते न च रोगाः स्युः शारीरागन्तुमानसाः।।
Praśastavāstuni gṛhē śucāvātapavarjitē
nivātē na ca rōgā: syu: śārīrāgantumānasā: SS. Sū: 19 – 4

5. The patient may distrust his mother, father, sons, and relatives but would put himself in the physician's hands with complete trust. The physician should therefore, safeguard him like his son.

मातरं पितरं पुत्रान् बान्धवानपि चातुरः।
अप्येतानभिशङ्केत वैद्यो विश्वासमेति च।।
विसृजत्यात्मनाऽऽत्मानं न चैनं परिशङ्कते।
तस्मात् पुत्रवदेवैनं पालयेदातुरं भिषक्।।
Mātaraṃ pitaraṃ putrān bāndhavānapi cātura:
apyētānabhiśaṅkēta vaidyō viśvāsamēti ca
Visṛjatyātmanāऽऽtmānaṃ na cainaṃ pariśaṅkatē
tasmāt putravadēvainaṃ pālayēdāturaṃ bhiṣak SS. 25. 43 – 44

6. The Atharvanas list 101 deaths of which one is timely and natural, while the others are externally caused and unnatural.

एकोत्तरं मृत्युशतमथर्वाणः प्रचक्षते।
तत्रैकः कालसंयुक्तः शेषा आगन्तवः स्मृताः।।
Ēkōttaraṃ mṛtyuśatamatharvāṇa: pracakṣatē
tatraika: kālasamyukta: śēṣā āgantava: smṛtā: SS. Sū: 34. 6

7. As a helmsman steers the boat in a river even without attendants, a good physician is ever capable on his own of carrying the patient safely through the course of illness.

   वैद्यस्तु गुणवानेकस्तारयेदातुरं सदा।
   प्लवं प्रतितरैर्हीनं कर्णधार इवांभसि।।
   Vaidyastu guṇavānēkastārayēdāturaṃ sadā
   pḷavaṃ pratitarairhīnaṃ karṇadhāra ivāmbhasi SS. Sū: 34. 18

8. Formation of parts and subparts is done by nature; fault and faultlessness thereof should be known to be caused by the unrighteous and righteous conduct of the foetus in a previous existence.

   अङ्गप्रत्यङ्गनिर्वृत्तिः स्वभावादेव जायते ।
   अङ्गप्रत्यङ्गनिर्वृत्तौ ये भवन्ति गुणागुणाः ।।
   ते ते गर्भस्य विज्ञेया धर्माधर्मनिमित्तजाः ।
   Aṅgapratyaṅganirvṛtti: svabhāvādēva jāyatē
   aṅgapratyaṅganirvṛttau yē bhavanti guṇāguṇā:
   Tē tē garbhasya vijñēyā dharmādharmanimittajā: SS. Śa: 3. 36

9. Activity, which exerts the whole body is physical exercise.

   शरीरायासजननं कर्म व्यायामसंज्ञितम् ।।
   Śarīrāyāsajananaṃ karma vyāyāmasamjñitaṃ SS. Ci: 24. 38

10. Vāta, pitta, and kapha are the three doṣas; in equilibrium, they sustain the body and in disequilibrium, destroy it.

    वायुः पित्तं कफश्चेति त्रयो दोषाः समासतः
    विकृताविकृता देहं घ्नन्ति ते वर्तयन्ति च
    Vāyuḥ pittam kaphaśceti trayo doṣāḥ samāsataḥ
    Vikṛtāvikṛtā deham ghnanti te vartayanti ca AH. Sūtra 1 – 6

11. A patient should be examined by inspection, touch, and interrogation.

    दर्शनस्पर्शनप्रश्नैः परीक्षेत च रोगिणम्
    Darśanasparśanapraśnaiḥ parīkṣeta ca rogiṇam AH Sūtra 1. 21

12. Lightness of the body, manual dexterity, vigorous digestion, reduction of fat, firm, and solid organs are the fruits of physical exercise.

लाघवं कर्मसामर्थ्यं दीप्तोऽग्निर्मेदसः क्षयः
विभक्तघनगात्रत्वं व्यायामादुपजायते
Lāghavam karmasāmarthyam dīptoऽgnirmedasaḥ kṣayaḥ
Vibhaktaghanagātratvam vyāyāmādupajāyate AH Sūtra 2. 10

13. Harming others, theft, sexual misconduct, slander, harsh speaking of untruth, divisive speech, malice, greed, and lack of faith are the ten sinful acts of the body, speech, and mind to be shunned.

हिंसास्तेयान्यथाकामं पैशून्यं परुषानृते
सम्भिन्नालापं व्यापादमभिध्यां दृग्विपर्ययम्
पापं कर्मेति दशधा कायवाङ्मानसैस्त्यजेत्
Himsāsteyānyathākāmam paiśūnyam paruṣānṛte
Sambhinnālāpam vyāpādamabhidhyām dṛgviparyayam
Pāpam karmeti daśadhā kāyavāṅmānasaistyajet AH Sūtra 2. 21 – 22

14. One should always regard even mites and ants as no different from oneself.

आत्मवत् सततं पश्येदपि कीटपिपीलिकाम्
Ātmavat satatam paśyedapi kīṭapipīlikām AH Sūtra: 2. 23

15. One should be of service even to an enemy who may be intent on doing harm.

उपकारप्रधानः स्यादपकारपरेऽप्यरौ
Upakārapradhānaḥ syādapakārapareऽpyarau AH Sūtra: 2. 24

16. One should speak timely, agreeably, briefly, truthfully, and gently.

काले हितं मितं ब्रूयादविसंवादि पेशलम्
Kāle hitam mitam brūyādavisamvādi peśalam AH Sūtra: 2. 25

17. In performing all work, one should adopt the middle path.

अनुयायात्प्रतिपदं सर्वधर्मेषु मध्यमाम्
Anuyāyātpratipadam sarvadharmeṣu madhyamām AH Sūtra: 2. 30

18. For the wise, the whole world is a teacher in all he does; therefore, as a man of action in the world's theatre, he should emulate its example.

आचार्यः सर्वचेष्टासु लोक एव हि धीमतः
अनुकुर्यात्तमेवातो लौकिकेऽर्थे परीक्षकः
Ācāryaḥ sarvaceṣṭāsu loka eva hi dhīmataḥ
Anukuryāttamevāto laukikeऽrthe parīkṣakaḥ AH Sūtra: 2. 45

19. Compassion for living creatures; charity; tamed body, speech, and mind; regarding others as one's own—these are the elements of virtuous conduct.

आर्द्रसन्तानता त्यागः कायवाक्चेतसां दमः
स्वार्थबुद्धिः परार्थेषु पर्याप्तमिति सद्व्रतम्
Ārdrasantānatā tyāgaḥ kāyavākcetasām damaḥ
Svārthabuddhiḥ parārtheṣu paryāptamiti sadvratam AH Sūtra: 2. 46

20. One who enjoys wholesome food and activity every day; who introspects on his actions; who is unattached; who is generous; who looks on all with an equal eye; who is truthful and forgiving; who delights in the service of the virtuous he remains free from illness.

नित्यं हिताहारविहारसेवी समीक्ष्यकारी विषयेष्वसक्तः
दाता समः सत्यपरः क्षमावानाप्तोपसेवी च भवत्यरोगः
Nityam hitāhāravihārasevī samīkṣyakārī viṣayeṣvasaktaḥ
Dātā samaḥ satyaparaḥ kṣamāvānāptopasevī ca bhavatyarogaḥ AH Sūtra: 4. 36

21. While eating a meal, half the stomach should be filled by solids; a quarter by liquids, and a quarter left for free airflow.

अन्नेन कुक्षेर्द्वावंशौ पानेनैकं प्रपूरयेत्
आश्रयं पवनादीनां चतुर्थमवशेषयेत्
Annena kukṣerdvāvamśau pānenaikam prapūrayet
Āśrayam pavanādīnām caturthamavaśeṣayet AH Sūtra: 8. 46

22. A physician should never feel ashamed of being unable to name a disease; the fact is that all diseases have not been named.

विकारनामाकुशलो न जिह्रीयात् कदाचन
न हि सर्वविकाराणां नामतोऽस्ति ध्रुवा स्थिति
Vikāranāmākuśalo na jihrīyāt kadācana
Na hi sarvavikārāṇām nāmatoऽsti dhruvā sthiti AH Sūtra: 12. 64

23. A person addicted to wine can hardly distinguish right from wrong; happiness from unhappiness; proper from improper and wholesome from unwholesome. How then could an enlightened individual take to addiction?

धर्माधर्मं सुखं दुःखमर्थानर्थं हिताहितम्
यदासक्तो न जानाति कथं तच्छीलयेद्बुधः
Dharmādharmam sukham duḥkhamarthānartham hitāhitam
Yadāsakto na jānāti katham tacchīlayedbudhaḥ AH Nidana: 6.8

24. A mind, pure and soaked in compassion, is the best febrifuge.

करुणार्द्रं मनः शुद्धं सर्वज्वरविनाशनम्
Karuṇārdram manaḥ śuddham sarvajvaravināśanam AH Cikitsa: 1. 73

25. Truthfulness; freedom from anger; self-control over senses; tranquility and adherence to a code of good conduct are indeed the everlasting rasāyana.

सत्यवादिनमक्रोधमध्यात्मप्रवणेन्द्रियम्
शान्तं सद्वृत्तनिरतं विद्यान्नित्यरसायनम्
Satyavādinamakrodhamadhyātmapravaṇendriyam
Śāntam sadvṛttaniratam vidyānnityarasāyanam AH Uttara: 39. 179

26. One should keep far away from the despicable physician who knows the medical texts by heart but has failed to grasp their true meaning.

अज्ञातशास्त्रसद्भान् शास्त्रमात्रपरायणान्
त्यजेद्दूरान् भिषक्पाशान् पाशान् वैवस्वतानिव
Ajñātaśāstrasadbhāvān śāstramātraparāyaṇān
Tyajeddūrān bhiṣakpāśān pāśān vaivasvatāniva AH Uttara: 40. 76

27. Glory to the physicians of noble conduct and keen understanding of medical texts. Glory to the physicians whose practical experience is profound. Glory to the physicians who regard all living beings as their own children and friends.

भिषजां साधुवृत्तानां भद्रमागमशालिनाम्
अभ्यस्तकर्मणां भद्रं भद्रं भद्राभिलाषिणाम्
Bhiṣajām sādhuvṛttānām bhadramāgamaśālinām
Abhyastakarmaṇām bhadram bhadram bhadrābhilāṣiṇām AH Uttara: 40. 77

28. Health is the basis of virtuous conduct, wealth, pursuit of happiness and spiritual liberation.

धर्मार्थकाममोक्षाणामारोग्यं मूलमुत्तमम् ।
Dharmārthakāmamokṣāṇāmārogyam mūlamuttamam CS. Sūtra: 1.15

29. The object of mind is what can be thought of

मनसस्तु चिन्त्यमर्थः
Manasastu cintyamarthaḥ CS. Sūtra: 1.16

30. All Internal disorders arising from body components (dhātus) are not separate from vāta, pitta and kapha; only external causes are separate.

स्वधातुवैषम्यनिमित्तजा ये
विकारसंघा बहवः शरीरे ।
न ते पृथक् पित्तकफानिलेभ्य
आगन्तवस्त्वेव ततो विशिष्टाः ।। CS. Sūtra: 20.6

Svadhātuvaiṣamyanimittajā ye
vikārasamghā bahavaḥ śarīre
Na te pṛthak pittakaphānilebhyaḥ
āgantavastveva tato viśiṣṭāḥ CS. Sūtra: 20.6

31. There was never a time when the unbroken flow of life or intellect did not exist: the knowers of Āyurveda are also eternal in so far as the procession of health and disease, causes and symptoms and their interactions are also eternal.

न हि नाभूत् कदाचिदायुषः सन्तानो बुद्धिसन्तानो वा,
शाश्वतश्चायुषो वेदिता, अनादि च सुखदुःखं
सद्रव्यहेतुलक्षणमपरापरयोगात्।

Na hi nābhūt kadācidāyuṣaḥ santāno buddhisantāno vā,
śāśvataścāyuṣo veditā, anādi ca
sukhaduḥkham sadravyahetulakṣaṇamaparāparayogāt CS. Sūtra: 30.27

32. The wrong actions carried out by those whose intellect, self-control and memory are unsettled are known as imprudent conduct (prajñāparādha) which deranges all doṣas.

धीधृतिस्मृतिविभ्रष्टः कर्म यत् कुरुतेऽशुभम्।
प्रज्ञापराधं तं विद्यात् सर्वदोषप्रकोपणम्।।

Dhīdhṛtismṛtivibhraṣṭaḥ karma yat kuruteऽśubham
Prajñāparādham tam vidyāt sarvadoṣaprakopaṇam CS. Śārīra: 1.102

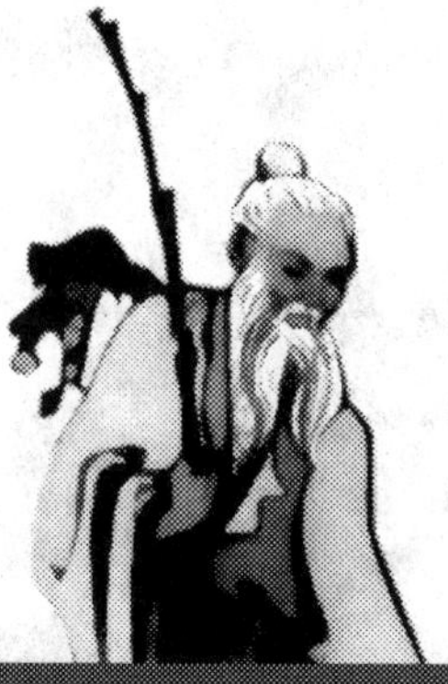

BOTANICAL NAMES

Plants	Botanical Names
Abhiṣuka	? Pistacia vera Linn.
Ādraka	Zingiber officinale Rosc. (fresh)
Ajagandhā	*Cleome viscosa* Linn.
Ākṣikī	*Terminalia bellirica (Gaertn.)* Roxb.
Alābū	*Lagenaria siceraria* (Mol.) Standley
Āmalaka	*Phyllanthus emblica* Linn.
Amlacāṅgērī	Oxalis corniculata Linn.
Amḷavetasa	*Solena amplexicaulis* (Lam.) Gandhi
Amlīkā	Tamarindus indica Linn.
Āmra	*Mangifera indica* Linn.
Āmrāta	Tinosporia cordifolia (Willd.) Hook. f & Thoms.
Āmṛātaka	*Spondias pinnata* (Linn. f.) Kurz
Amrtā	*Tinospora cordifolia* (Willd.) Miers ex Hook.f. & Thoms.
Aṅkoṭa	*Alangium salvifolium* (Linn.f.) Wang
Aśvattha	*Ficus religiosa* Linn.
Bākucī	*Psoralea corylifolia* Linn.
Balā	*Sida rhombifolia* Linn. ssp. *retusa* (Linn.) Borssum
Bhallātaka	*Semecarpus anacardium* Linn.
Bhandī	Albīzia lebbeck (Linn.) Benth.
Bhavya	*Dillenia indica* Linn.
Bhūṣṭṛṇa	*Cymbopogon citratus* (DC.) Stapf
Bibhītaka	*Terminalia bellirica* (Gaertn.) Roxb.
Bilva	*Aegle marmelos* (Linn.) Corr.
Bilvaparṇī	Limonia crenulata Roxb.?
Bimbī	*Coccinia grandis* (Linn.) Voigt.

Plants	Botanical Names
Cakramarda	*Cassia tora* Linn.
Citraka	*Plumbago zeylanica* L.
Dāḍima	*Punica granatum* Linn.
Dantaśatha	*Citrus limon* (Linn.) Burm.f.
Dantī	*Baliospermum montanum* (Willd.) Muell. -Arg.
Dhānyaka	*Coriandrum sativum* Linn.
Eraṇḍa	*Ricinus communis* Linn.
Ervāruka	*Cucumis melo* var. *utilissimus* (Roxb.) Duthie &
Gaṇḍīra	*Cayratia trifolia* (L.) Domin
Gandīra	*Cayratia carnosa* (Wall. ex Wight.) Gagnep.
Gāṅgerukī	Sida cordata (Burm.f.) Borssum
Gṛñjanaka	*Allium ascalonicum* L.
Iṅgudī	*Sarcostigma kleinii* Wight & Arn.
Jalapippalī	Phyla nodiflora Linn. (Lippia nodiflora (Linn.) A. Rich.)
Jambīra	*Citrus limon* (Linn.) Burm.f.
Jambū	*Syzygium cumini* (Linn.) Skeels
Jīvantī	*Holostemma ada-kodien* Schultes
Jujube (Kōlāmla)	Zizyphus mauritiana Lam.
Kākamācī	*Solanum nigrum* Linn.
Kāḷaśāka	*Corchorus capsularis* L.
Kalāya	*Pisum sativum* Linn.
Kapittha	*Limonia acidissima* L.
Karañja	*Pongamia pinnata* (Linn.) Merr.
Karbudāra	*Bauhinia purpurea* L./Bauhinia variegata Linn.
Karcūra	Curcuma zedoaria Rosc.
Karīra	*Capparis decidua* Edgew.
Kāsamarda	*Senna occidentalis* (L.) Link
Kāśmarya	Gmelina arbeorea Linn.
Kelūṭa	Brassica oleracea Linn. var. capitata Linn.
Kembuka	*Brassica oleracea* L. var. *capitata* L.
Ketakī	*Pandanus odoratissimus* Roxb.
Kovidāra	*Bauhinia purpurea* Linn.
Krauñcādana	Nelumbo nucifera Gaertn. (Petiole)

Plants	Botanical Names
Kumārajīva	Drypetes roxburghii (Wall.) Huresawa (Putranjiva roxburghii Wall)
Kūśmāṇḍa	*Benincasa hispida* (Thunb.) Cobn.
Kūśmāṇḍaka	Benincasa hispida (Thunb.) Cogn.
Kusumbhā	*Carthamus tinctorius* Linn.
Kuṭumbaka	Cymbopogon citratus (DC.) Stapf
Lāṅgalikā	Gloriosa superba Linn.
Laśuna	*Allium sativum* Linn.
Lavalī	*Cicca acida* (Linn.) Merrill
Maṇḍūkaparṇī	*Centella asiatica* (Linn.) Urban.
Moca	*Musa paradisiaca* Linn.
Mūlaka	*Raphanus sativus* Linn.
Muñjātaka	Orchis latifolia Linn.
Nāgaraṅga	Citrus reticulata Blanco
Nārīkela	*Cocos nucifera* Linn.
Nimba	*Azadirachta indica* A.Juss.
Nīpa	*Mytragyna parviflora* Korth.
Niṣpāva	*Lablab purpureus* Linn.
Palāṇḍu	*Allium cepa* Linn.
Panasa	*Artocarpus heterophyllus* Linn.
Pārāvata	*Garcinia cowa* Roxb.
Parūṣaka	*Grewia asiatica* Linn.
Pāṭhā (Kucēlā)	Cissampelos pariera Linn.
Pīlu	*Salvadora persica* Linn. var. *wightiana* Verdc.
Rājādana	*Manilkara hexandra* (Roxb.) Dubard
Rājakṣavaka	*Brassica nigra* (L.) Koch.
Śaṇa	*Crotalaria retusa* Linn.
Śatāvarī	*Asparagus racemosus* Willd.
Śatī	*Hedychium spicatum* Ham. ex Smith
Śigru	*Moringa oleifera* Lam./*Moringa pterygosperma* Gaertn.
Śimbītakā	Lablab purpureus Linn. (Dolichos lablab Linn.)
Śḷeṣmātaka	*Cordia dichotoma* Forster
Śreyasī (Gajapippalī)	*Scindapsus officinalis* (Roxb.) Schott
Śreyasī (Rāsnā)	*Alpinia galanga* (L.) Willd.

Plants	Botanical Names
Surasā	*Ocimum tenuiflorum* Linn.
Tāla	*Borassus flabellifer* Linn.
Tālapralambha	Borassus flabellifer Linn.
Taṇḍulīya	*Amaranthus spinosus* L.
Taṅka	Pyrus communis Linn.
Tarūṭa	Nymphaea Sp. (Rhizome)
Tila	*Sesamum indicum* Linn.
Tinḍuka	*Diospyros malabarica* (Desr.) Kostel.
Trapusā	*Cucumis sativus* Linn.
Triparṇī	Uraria lagopoides (Linn.) Desv.
Uḍumbara	*Ficus racemosa* Linn.
Upodikā	*Basella alba* var. *rubra* (Linn.) Stewart
Utpala	*Nymphaea alba* Linn.
Vārtāka	*Solanum melongena* Linn.
Vāstuka	*Chenopodium album* Linn.
Vātāma	Prunus amygdalus Baill.
Vatsādanī	*Tinospora cordifolia* (Willd.) Miers ex Hook.f. & Thoms.
Vētasa	*Homonoia riparia* Lour.
Vidārīkaṇḍa	Pueraria tuberosa DC.
Vṛkṣāṃḷa	Garcinia indica Chois.
Yavānī	*Trachyspermum ammi* (Linn.) Sprague

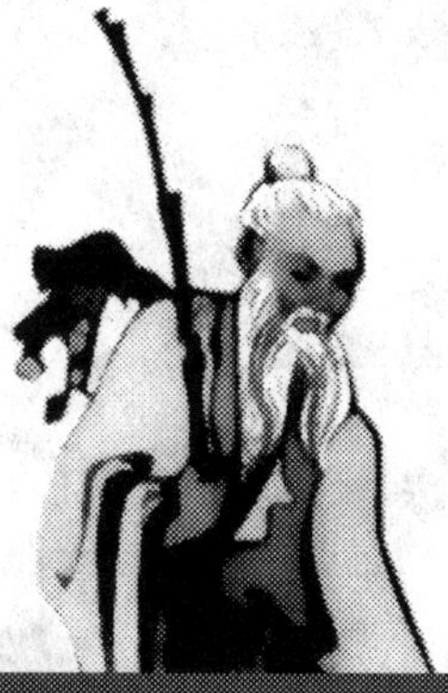

GLOSSARY

Ādāna	Lean half of the year
Ādhibhautika	Illness due to external events like storms, floods
Ādhidaivika	Illness as a consequence of fate or wrath of gods
Ādhyatmika	Illness due to perturbed doṣas
Agada	Toxicology: Branch of Āyurveda
Agni	Fire; one of pañcabhūtas
Agnikarma	Thermal cautery
Agniveśa	Disciple of Ātreya: Author of a tantra which was redacted by Caraka
Āhārarasa	Rasa, assimilable part of digested food
Ākāśa	Ether; one of pañcabhūtas
Alābu	A vessel made of gourd
Amḷa	Sour
Anumāna	Inference
Ap	Water; one of pañcabhūtas
Apta	Moral and scholarly authority
Āśrama	A residential school
Aṣṭaṅga	Eight branches of Āyurveda
Ātreya	Patron saint of Āyurveda; teacher of Agniveśa
Āturavṛtta	Care of the ill
Bhagandara	Anorectal fistula
Bhikku	A Buddhist mendicant
Bhūta	Elements
Bhūtavidyā	Treatment of mental disorders

Bimbisāra	Mauryan emperor: father of Ashoka
Brāhmaṇa	Section of the Vedas dealing with rules for performing rituals
Bṛhattrayī	Great three (Caraka, Suśruta and Vāgbhaṭa)
Buddhaghoṣa	Great Buddhist scholar, author of Visuddhimagga
Caraka	Author of Caraka Samhita and physician-extraordinary
Cetana	Consciousness
Daiva	Fate
Dhamani	A type of body conduits
Dhātu	Body tissue
Dinacarya	Daily routine for a healthy life
Dīpana	Digestion;
Divodāsa	King of Kāśi, acclaimed as an incarnation of Dhanvantari
Dravya	Substance
Gorasa	Milk and milk products
Gurukula	A traditional method of education where the disciples stayed with the teacher
Harita	Green vegetables in diet
Ikṣu	Sugar
Indriya	Senses of perception and action
Jaḷauka	Leeches
Janapadodhwamsana	Destruction of habitat
Jentaka	Body fomentation in a special chamber
Jīvaka	Celebrated physician of the Buddha; surgeon
Kanāda	Pioneer of Vaiśeṣika system of Indian philosophy
Kaniṣka	Famed emperor of Kuṣāna period
Kapha	One of the three doṣas
Karma	Law of past actions producing later effects
Kaṣāya	Astringent
Kaṭu	Pungent
Kāyacikitsa	Branch of Āyurveda dealing with internal medicine
Kitta	Execrable part resulting from digestion of food in the gut

Kriyākāla	Stages in the progression of disease
Kṣāra	Alkali
Kuṭipraveśika	Indoor variety of rejuvenation therapy
Lavaṇa	Salty
Madhura	Sweet
Madya	Liquor/wine
Mahasrotas	Alimentary canal
Māmsa	Muscle
Manas	Mind
Marma	Vital spot
Nādīyantra	Tubular instrument
Nāgārjuna	Scholar who redacted Suśruta Samhita in 4th century CE
Nasya	Nasal purging
Nyāya sūtra	The text of the Nyāya system of philosophy, attributed to Gautama
Pañcabhūta	Five elements of which the universe is composed
Pariṇāma	Evolution
Pariṣad	Assembly
Phala	Fruits
Pitta	One of the three doṣas
Pittala	Pitta prone constitution
Prabhāva	Action of drugs – beyond taste, potency and post-digestive taste
Prajñāparādha	Error of judgment with imprudent conduct
Prakṛti	Body constitution; nature
Prāṇa	A division of vāta; vital breath
Pratyakṣa	Perception as a valid source of knowledge
Pṛthvī	Earth; one of pañcabhūtas
Rajas	Second mental quality marked by activity
Rājasa	Possessing the quality of Rajas
Rakta visrāvaṇa	Blood letting
Rasa	Taste; assimilable part of digested food

Rasāyana	Rejuvenant therapy
Riṣṭa	Signs of impending death
Roga	Disease
Ṛtucarya	Seasonal regimen for a healthy life
Sabda	Authoritative testimony
Sadvṛtti	Virtuous conduct
Śāka	Vegetable
Śalāka	Rod like instrument
Śālākya	Head and neck disorders
Śalya	Branch of Āyurveda dealing with surgery; foreign body in the body issues
Śamana	Pacification of perturbed doṣas
Sambhāṣa	Discussion for learning
Śamīdhānya	Pulses
Sāmya	Equilibrium
Sangha	Buddhist fraternity
Sāṅkhya	One of the six systems of Indian philosophy
Śastṛa	Sharp instrument
Siddha	Traditional medicine of India practiced in Tamil Nadu
Sira	Body channel / vein
Śira	Head
Sleṣmala	Kapha prone constitution
Snehana	Lubricant therapy
Śodhana	Evacuative therapy
Śṛṅga	Animal horn used for suction
Srotas	Channels/ conduits in the body
Śūkadhānya	Husked grains
Suśruta	Pioneer of Surgery in Āyurveda: author of Suśruta Samhita
Svasthavṛtta	Healthy life / Protection of health
Svastika	Instruments where two arms cross like scissors: forceps
Svedana	Fomentation

Takṣaśila	Ancient University noted for medical studies – (modern Taxila in Pakistan)
Talayantra	Spoon-shaped instruments
Tamas	Third mental quality marked by inertia
Tāmasa	Possessing the quality of tamas
Tikta	Bitter
Tridoṣa	Three products of digestive process in the body: crucial to health and disease
Vāgbhaṭa	Author of Aṣṭāṅgahṛdaya; poet
Vaiśeṣika	One of the six systems of Indian philosophy
Vājīkaraṇa	Enhancement of potency
Vamana	Emesis
Vasti	Enema
Vāta	One of the three doṣas
Vātala	Vata prone constitution
Vātātapika	Open air variety of rejuvenant therapy
Vāyu	Air; one of pañcabhūtas
Vedanta	One of the six systems of Indian philosophy
Vipāka	Post-digestive taste of food and drugs
Virecana	Purgation
Vīrya	Potency
Visarga	Generous half of the year
Yantra	Blunt instrument
Yoga	One of the six systems of Indian philosophy
Yukti	Reason

Printed in the United States
by Baker & Taylor Publisher Services